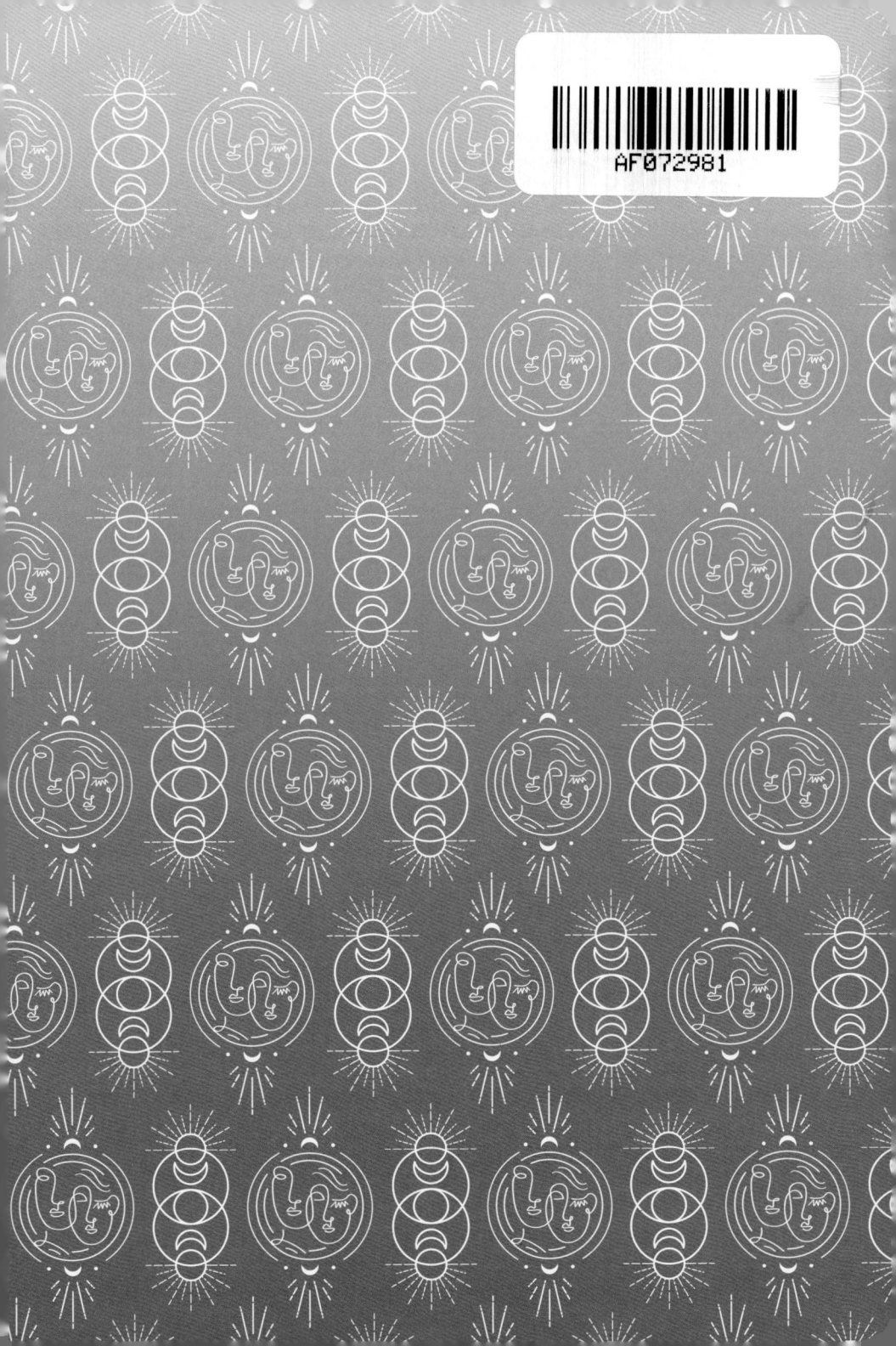

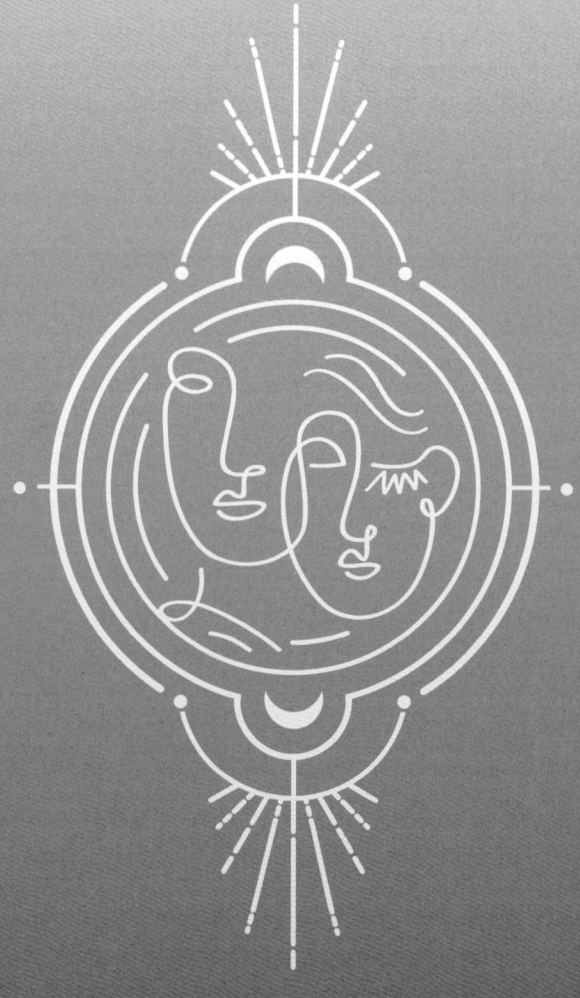

THIS JOURNAL BELONGS TO:

_____

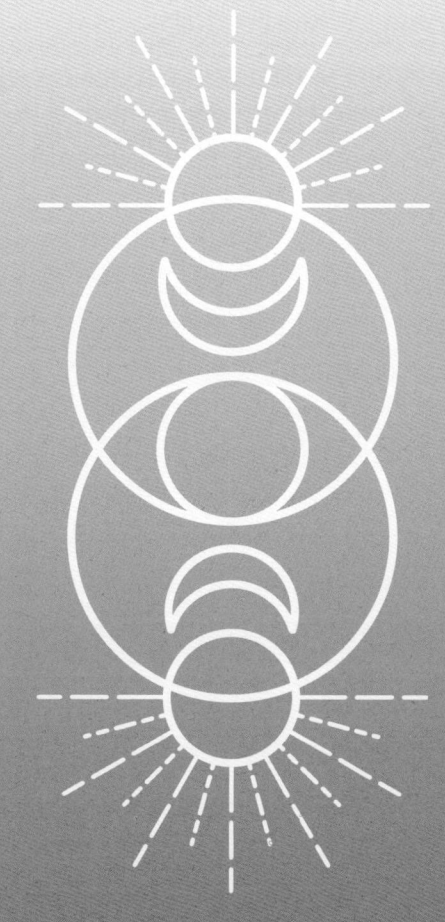

CONNECTION

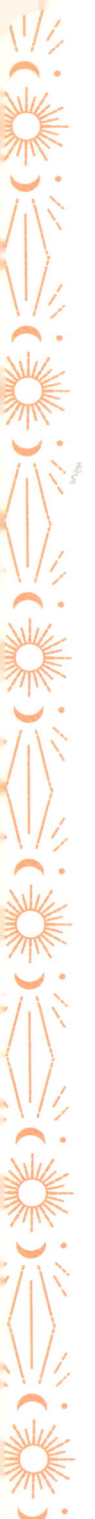
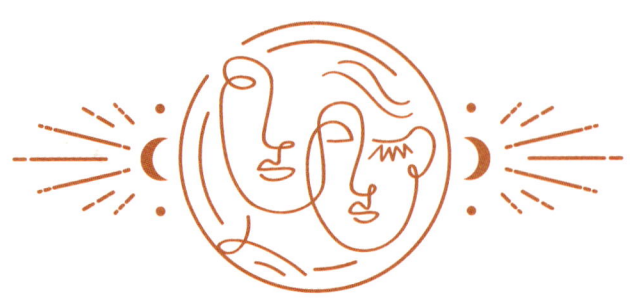

Deep, personal connections are good for your mind, body, and soul, and are at the core of some of our most essential needs as humans. Cultivating strong connections can positively benefit your health, increase your longevity, keep your mind engaged and sharp, and inspire passion and creativity. It is not the quantity of your connections but the quality of these deeper bonds that matter and give your life meaning.

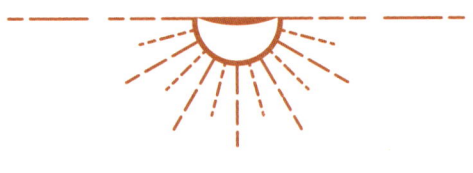

This 90-day journal supports your daily, intentional efforts to establish and maintain meaningful connections with family, friends, and yourself. Each day is divided into two sections, "Record" and "Reflect." The first section is a place for you to record your goals and actions. The second section provides an opportunity to reflect on how your efforts throughout the day contributed to your overall feelings of connectedness. In addition, this journal includes three monthly "Connection Calendars" that allow you the space to plan and set reminders for the deeper bonds you want to make.

With this journal as your guide, you will learn to set intentions and reflect on actions that will help to improve your ability to cultivate fulfilling connections in your life.

CONNECTION CALENDAR
EVENTS, PLANS, AND GOALS FOR CONNECTING THIS MONTH

MONDAY	TUESDAY	WEDNESDAY	THURSDAY

MONTH: _____   YEAR: _____

FRIDAY	SATURDAY	SUNDAY

NOTES:

CONNECTION CALENDAR
EVENTS, PLANS, AND GOALS FOR CONNECTING THIS MONTH

MONDAY	TUESDAY	WEDNESDAY	THURSDAY

MONTH: _____   YEAR: _____

FRIDAY	SATURDAY	SUNDAY

NOTES:

CONNECTION CALENDAR
EVENTS, PLANS, AND GOALS FOR CONNECTING THIS MONTH

MONDAY	TUESDAY	WEDNESDAY	THURSDAY

MONTH: _____ YEAR: _____

FRIDAY	SATURDAY	SUNDAY

NOTES:

RECORD

DATE ___/___/___

MY GOALS FOR MEANINGFUL CONNECTIONS TODAY:

- [ ] _____
- [ ] _____
- [ ] _____

PEOPLE I'D LIKE TO CONNECT WITH:
_____
_____

WAYS TO STRENGTHEN MY RELATIONSHIPS:
_____
_____

WAYS I CONNECTED WITH OTHERS TODAY:

- [ ] CALLED A FRIEND
- [ ] ENCOURAGED SOMEONE
- [ ] ASKED FOR HELP OR ADVICE
- [ ] PLANNED ONE-ON-ONE TIME
- [ ] PRACTICED ACTIVE LISTENING
- [ ] EXPRESSED MY GRATITUDE TO SOMEONE ELSE
- [ ] SPENT QUALITY TIME WITH A FRIEND OR FAMILY MEMBER
- [ ] HELPED SOMEONE
- [ ] SHARED SOMETHING PERSONAL ABOUT MYSELF
- [ ] PRACTICED VULNERABILITY WITH A TRUSTED FRIEND
- [ ] SHARED A LAUGH
- [ ] TALKED TO SOMEONE NEW
- [ ] COMPLIMENTED SOMEONE
- [ ] COMPLETED A SHARED ACTIVITY
- [ ] NOTED SOMEONE ELSE'S MEANINGFUL DATE, EVENT, OR INTEREST I'D LIKE TO REMEMBER
- [ ] LET SOMEONE KNOW I WAS THINKING OF THEM
- [ ] PRACTICED BEING MORE PRESENT WITH OTHERS
- [ ] SHARED A STORY
- [ ] WROTE A PERSONAL NOTE OR TEXT

REFLECT

HOW I'D RATE MY FEELING OF CONNECTION TODAY:

| 1 | 2 | 3 | 4 | 5 | 6 | 7 | 8 | 9 | 10 |

LONELY / DISCONNECTED　　　　　　　　　　　　　　　　HIGHLY CONNECTED

THE MOST MEANINGFUL INTERACTION I HAD TODAY AND HOW IT MADE ME FEEL:

_____
_____
_____
_____
_____
_____
_____
_____

CHALLENGES TO DEVELOPING DEEPER BONDS AND HOW I CAN OVERCOME THEM:

_____
_____
_____
_____

WAYS I'D LIKE TO CONNECT MORE:

_____
_____
_____
_____
_____

RECORD

DATE ___/___/___

MY GOALS FOR MEANINGFUL CONNECTIONS TODAY:

- [ ] _____
- [ ] _____
- [ ] _____

PEOPLE I'D LIKE TO CONNECT WITH:

_____
_____

WAYS TO STRENGTHEN MY RELATIONSHIPS:

_____
_____

WAYS I CONNECTED WITH OTHERS TODAY:

- [ ] CALLED A FRIEND
- [ ] ENCOURAGED SOMEONE
- [ ] ASKED FOR HELP OR ADVICE
- [ ] PLANNED ONE-ON-ONE TIME
- [ ] PRACTICED ACTIVE LISTENING
- [ ] EXPRESSED MY GRATITUDE TO SOMEONE ELSE
- [ ] SPENT QUALITY TIME WITH A FRIEND OR FAMILY MEMBER
- [ ] HELPED SOMEONE
- [ ] SHARED SOMETHING PERSONAL ABOUT MYSELF
- [ ] PRACTICED VULNERABILITY WITH A TRUSTED FRIEND
- [ ] SHARED A LAUGH
- [ ] TALKED TO SOMEONE NEW
- [ ] COMPLIMENTED SOMEONE
- [ ] COMPLETED A SHARED ACTIVITY
- [ ] NOTED SOMEONE ELSE'S MEANINGFUL DATE, EVENT, OR INTEREST I'D LIKE TO REMEMBER
- [ ] LET SOMEONE KNOW I WAS THINKING OF THEM
- [ ] PRACTICED BEING MORE PRESENT WITH OTHERS
- [ ] SHARED A STORY
- [ ] WROTE A PERSONAL NOTE OR TEXT

REFLECT

HOW I'D RATE MY FEELING OF CONNECTION TODAY:

| 1 | 2 | 3 | 4 | 5 | 6 | 7 | 8 | 9 | 10 |

LONELY / DISCONNECTED   HIGHLY CONNECTED

THE MOST MEANINGFUL INTERACTION I HAD TODAY AND HOW IT MADE ME FEEL:

_____
_____
_____
_____
_____
_____
_____
_____

CHALLENGES TO DEVELOPING DEEPER BONDS AND HOW I CAN OVERCOME THEM:

_____
_____
_____
_____

WAYS I'D LIKE TO CONNECT MORE:

_____
_____
_____
_____
_____

RECORD

DATE ___/___/___

MY GOALS FOR MEANINGFUL CONNECTIONS TODAY:

- [ ] _____
- [ ] _____
- [ ] _____

PEOPLE I'D LIKE TO CONNECT WITH:
_____
_____

WAYS TO STRENGTHEN MY RELATIONSHIPS:
_____
_____

WAYS I CONNECTED WITH OTHERS TODAY:

- [ ] CALLED A FRIEND
- [ ] ENCOURAGED SOMEONE
- [ ] ASKED FOR HELP OR ADVICE
- [ ] PLANNED ONE-ON-ONE TIME
- [ ] PRACTICED ACTIVE LISTENING
- [ ] EXPRESSED MY GRATITUDE TO SOMEONE ELSE
- [ ] SPENT QUALITY TIME WITH A FRIEND OR FAMILY MEMBER
- [ ] HELPED SOMEONE
- [ ] SHARED SOMETHING PERSONAL ABOUT MYSELF
- [ ] PRACTICED VULNERABILITY WITH A TRUSTED FRIEND
- [ ] SHARED A LAUGH
- [ ] TALKED TO SOMEONE NEW
- [ ] COMPLIMENTED SOMEONE
- [ ] COMPLETED A SHARED ACTIVITY
- [ ] NOTED SOMEONE ELSE'S MEANINGFUL DATE, EVENT, OR INTEREST I'D LIKE TO REMEMBER
- [ ] LET SOMEONE KNOW I WAS THINKING OF THEM
- [ ] PRACTICED BEING MORE PRESENT WITH OTHERS
- [ ] SHARED A STORY
- [ ] WROTE A PERSONAL NOTE OR TEXT

REFLECT

HOW I'D RATE MY FEELING OF CONNECTION TODAY:

| 1 | 2 | 3 | 4 | 5 | 6 | 7 | 8 | 9 | 10 |

LONELY / DISCONNECTED   HIGHLY CONNECTED

THE MOST MEANINGFUL INTERACTION I HAD TODAY AND HOW IT MADE ME FEEL:

CHALLENGES TO DEVELOPING DEEPER BONDS AND HOW I CAN OVERCOME THEM:

WAYS I'D LIKE TO CONNECT MORE:

RECORD

DATE ___/___/___

MY GOALS FOR MEANINGFUL CONNECTIONS TODAY:

- [ ] _____
- [ ] _____
- [ ] _____

PEOPLE I'D LIKE TO CONNECT WITH:

_____
_____

WAYS TO STRENGTHEN MY RELATIONSHIPS:

_____
_____

WAYS I CONNECTED WITH OTHERS TODAY:

- [ ] CALLED A FRIEND
- [ ] ENCOURAGED SOMEONE
- [ ] ASKED FOR HELP OR ADVICE
- [ ] PLANNED ONE-ON-ONE TIME
- [ ] PRACTICED ACTIVE LISTENING
- [ ] EXPRESSED MY GRATITUDE TO SOMEONE ELSE
- [ ] SPENT QUALITY TIME WITH A FRIEND OR FAMILY MEMBER
- [ ] HELPED SOMEONE
- [ ] SHARED SOMETHING PERSONAL ABOUT MYSELF
- [ ] PRACTICED VULNERABILITY WITH A TRUSTED FRIEND
- [ ] SHARED A LAUGH
- [ ] TALKED TO SOMEONE NEW
- [ ] COMPLIMENTED SOMEONE
- [ ] COMPLETED A SHARED ACTIVITY
- [ ] NOTED SOMEONE ELSE'S MEANINGFUL DATE, EVENT, OR INTEREST I'D LIKE TO REMEMBER
- [ ] LET SOMEONE KNOW I WAS THINKING OF THEM
- [ ] PRACTICED BEING MORE PRESENT WITH OTHERS
- [ ] SHARED A STORY
- [ ] WROTE A PERSONAL NOTE OR TEXT

REFLECT

HOW I'D RATE MY FEELING OF CONNECTION TODAY:

| 1 | 2 | 3 | 4 | 5 | 6 | 7 | 8 | 9 | 10 |

LONELY / DISCONNECTED   HIGHLY CONNECTED

THE MOST MEANINGFUL INTERACTION I HAD TODAY AND HOW IT MADE ME FEEL:

CHALLENGES TO DEVELOPING DEEPER BONDS AND HOW I CAN OVERCOME THEM:

WAYS I'D LIKE TO CONNECT MORE:

RECORD

DATE ___/___/___

MY GOALS FOR MEANINGFUL CONNECTIONS TODAY:

- ☐ _____
- ☐ _____
- ☐ _____

PEOPLE I'D LIKE TO CONNECT WITH:

_____
_____

WAYS TO STRENGTHEN MY RELATIONSHIPS:

_____
_____

WAYS I CONNECTED WITH OTHERS TODAY:

- ☐ CALLED A FRIEND
- ☐ ENCOURAGED SOMEONE
- ☐ ASKED FOR HELP OR ADVICE
- ☐ PLANNED ONE-ON-ONE TIME
- ☐ PRACTICED ACTIVE LISTENING
- ☐ EXPRESSED MY GRATITUDE TO SOMEONE ELSE
- ☐ SPENT QUALITY TIME WITH A FRIEND OR FAMILY MEMBER
- ☐ HELPED SOMEONE
- ☐ SHARED SOMETHING PERSONAL ABOUT MYSELF
- ☐ PRACTICED VULNERABILITY WITH A TRUSTED FRIEND
- ☐ SHARED A LAUGH
- ☐ TALKED TO SOMEONE NEW
- ☐ COMPLIMENTED SOMEONE
- ☐ COMPLETED A SHARED ACTIVITY
- ☐ NOTED SOMEONE ELSE'S MEANINGFUL DATE, EVENT, OR INTEREST I'D LIKE TO REMEMBER
- ☐ LET SOMEONE KNOW I WAS THINKING OF THEM
- ☐ PRACTICED BEING MORE PRESENT WITH OTHERS
- ☐ SHARED A STORY
- ☐ WROTE A PERSONAL NOTE OR TEXT

REFLECT

HOW I'D RATE MY FEELING OF CONNECTION TODAY:

| 1 | 2 | 3 | 4 | 5 | 6 | 7 | 8 | 9 | 10 |

LONELY / DISCONNECTED   HIGHLY CONNECTED

THE MOST MEANINGFUL INTERACTION I HAD TODAY AND HOW IT MADE ME FEEL:

___

CHALLENGES TO DEVELOPING DEEPER BONDS AND HOW I CAN OVERCOME THEM:

___

WAYS I'D LIKE TO CONNECT MORE:

___

RECORD

DATE ___/___/___

MY GOALS FOR MEANINGFUL CONNECTIONS TODAY:
- ☐ _____
- ☐ _____
- ☐ _____

PEOPLE I'D LIKE TO CONNECT WITH:
_____
_____

WAYS TO STRENGTHEN MY RELATIONSHIPS:
_____
_____

WAYS I CONNECTED WITH OTHERS TODAY:

- ☐ CALLED A FRIEND
- ☐ ENCOURAGED SOMEONE
- ☐ ASKED FOR HELP OR ADVICE
- ☐ PLANNED ONE-ON-ONE TIME
- ☐ PRACTICED ACTIVE LISTENING
- ☐ EXPRESSED MY GRATITUDE TO SOMEONE ELSE
- ☐ SPENT QUALITY TIME WITH A FRIEND OR FAMILY MEMBER
- ☐ HELPED SOMEONE
- ☐ SHARED SOMETHING PERSONAL ABOUT MYSELF
- ☐ PRACTICED VULNERABILITY WITH A TRUSTED FRIEND
- ☐ SHARED A LAUGH
- ☐ TALKED TO SOMEONE NEW
- ☐ COMPLIMENTED SOMEONE
- ☐ COMPLETED A SHARED ACTIVITY
- ☐ NOTED SOMEONE ELSE'S MEANINGFUL DATE, EVENT, OR INTEREST I'D LIKE TO REMEMBER
- ☐ LET SOMEONE KNOW I WAS THINKING OF THEM
- ☐ PRACTICED BEING MORE PRESENT WITH OTHERS
- ☐ SHARED A STORY
- ☐ WROTE A PERSONAL NOTE OR TEXT

REFLECT

HOW I'D RATE MY FEELING OF CONNECTION TODAY:

1	2	3	4	5	6	7	8	9	10

LONELY / DISCONNECTED   HIGHLY CONNECTED

THE MOST MEANINGFUL INTERACTION I HAD TODAY AND HOW IT MADE ME FEEL:

_____
_____
_____
_____
_____
_____
_____
_____

CHALLENGES TO DEVELOPING DEEPER BONDS AND HOW I CAN OVERCOME THEM:

_____
_____
_____
_____

WAYS I'D LIKE TO CONNECT MORE:

_____
_____
_____
_____

RECORD

DATE ___/___/___

MY GOALS FOR MEANINGFUL CONNECTIONS TODAY:

- [ ] _____
- [ ] _____
- [ ] _____

PEOPLE I'D LIKE TO CONNECT WITH:
_____
_____

WAYS TO STRENGTHEN MY RELATIONSHIPS:
_____
_____

WAYS I CONNECTED WITH OTHERS TODAY:

- [ ] CALLED A FRIEND
- [ ] ENCOURAGED SOMEONE
- [ ] ASKED FOR HELP OR ADVICE
- [ ] PLANNED ONE-ON-ONE TIME
- [ ] PRACTICED ACTIVE LISTENING
- [ ] EXPRESSED MY GRATITUDE TO SOMEONE ELSE
- [ ] SPENT QUALITY TIME WITH A FRIEND OR FAMILY MEMBER
- [ ] HELPED SOMEONE
- [ ] SHARED SOMETHING PERSONAL ABOUT MYSELF
- [ ] PRACTICED VULNERABILITY WITH A TRUSTED FRIEND
- [ ] SHARED A LAUGH
- [ ] TALKED TO SOMEONE NEW
- [ ] COMPLIMENTED SOMEONE
- [ ] COMPLETED A SHARED ACTIVITY
- [ ] NOTED SOMEONE ELSE'S MEANINGFUL DATE, EVENT, OR INTEREST I'D LIKE TO REMEMBER
- [ ] LET SOMEONE KNOW I WAS THINKING OF THEM
- [ ] PRACTICED BEING MORE PRESENT WITH OTHERS
- [ ] SHARED A STORY
- [ ] WROTE A PERSONAL NOTE OR TEXT

REFLECT

HOW I'D RATE MY FEELING OF CONNECTION TODAY:

| 1 | 2 | 3 | 4 | 5 | 6 | 7 | 8 | 9 | 10 |

LONELY / DISCONNECTED — HIGHLY CONNECTED

THE MOST MEANINGFUL INTERACTION I HAD TODAY AND HOW IT MADE ME FEEL:

CHALLENGES TO DEVELOPING DEEPER BONDS AND HOW I CAN OVERCOME THEM:

WAYS I'D LIKE TO CONNECT MORE:

RECORD

DATE ___/___/___

MY GOALS FOR MEANINGFUL CONNECTIONS TODAY:
- ☐ _____
- ☐ _____
- ☐ _____

PEOPLE I'D LIKE TO CONNECT WITH:
_____
_____

WAYS TO STRENGTHEN MY RELATIONSHIPS:
_____
_____

WAYS I CONNECTED WITH OTHERS TODAY:

- ☐ CALLED A FRIEND
- ☐ ENCOURAGED SOMEONE
- ☐ ASKED FOR HELP OR ADVICE
- ☐ PLANNED ONE-ON-ONE TIME
- ☐ PRACTICED ACTIVE LISTENING
- ☐ EXPRESSED MY GRATITUDE TO SOMEONE ELSE
- ☐ SPENT QUALITY TIME WITH A FRIEND OR FAMILY MEMBER
- ☐ HELPED SOMEONE
- ☐ SHARED SOMETHING PERSONAL ABOUT MYSELF
- ☐ PRACTICED VULNERABILITY WITH A TRUSTED FRIEND

- ☐ SHARED A LAUGH
- ☐ TALKED TO SOMEONE NEW
- ☐ COMPLIMENTED SOMEONE
- ☐ COMPLETED A SHARED ACTIVITY
- ☐ NOTED SOMEONE ELSE'S MEANINGFUL DATE, EVENT, OR INTEREST I'D LIKE TO REMEMBER
- ☐ LET SOMEONE KNOW I WAS THINKING OF THEM
- ☐ PRACTICED BEING MORE PRESENT WITH OTHERS
- ☐ SHARED A STORY
- ☐ WROTE A PERSONAL NOTE OR TEXT

REFLECT

HOW I'D RATE MY FEELING OF CONNECTION TODAY:

| 1 | 2 | 3 | 4 | 5 | 6 | 7 | 8 | 9 | 10 |

LONELY / DISCONNECTED   HIGHLY CONNECTED

THE MOST MEANINGFUL INTERACTION I HAD TODAY AND HOW IT MADE ME FEEL:

_____
_____
_____
_____
_____
_____
_____
_____

CHALLENGES TO DEVELOPING DEEPER BONDS AND HOW I CAN OVERCOME THEM:

_____
_____
_____
_____

WAYS I'D LIKE TO CONNECT MORE:

_____
_____
_____
_____

RECORD

DATE ___/___/___

MY GOALS FOR MEANINGFUL CONNECTIONS TODAY:

- [ ] _____
- [ ] _____
- [ ] _____

PEOPLE I'D LIKE TO CONNECT WITH:

_____
_____

WAYS TO STRENGTHEN MY RELATIONSHIPS:

_____
_____

WAYS I CONNECTED WITH OTHERS TODAY:

- [ ] CALLED A FRIEND
- [ ] ENCOURAGED SOMEONE
- [ ] ASKED FOR HELP OR ADVICE
- [ ] PLANNED ONE-ON-ONE TIME
- [ ] PRACTICED ACTIVE LISTENING
- [ ] EXPRESSED MY GRATITUDE TO SOMEONE ELSE
- [ ] SPENT QUALITY TIME WITH A FRIEND OR FAMILY MEMBER
- [ ] HELPED SOMEONE
- [ ] SHARED SOMETHING PERSONAL ABOUT MYSELF
- [ ] PRACTICED VULNERABILITY WITH A TRUSTED FRIEND
- [ ] SHARED A LAUGH
- [ ] TALKED TO SOMEONE NEW
- [ ] COMPLIMENTED SOMEONE
- [ ] COMPLETED A SHARED ACTIVITY
- [ ] NOTED SOMEONE ELSE'S MEANINGFUL DATE, EVENT, OR INTEREST I'D LIKE TO REMEMBER
- [ ] LET SOMEONE KNOW I WAS THINKING OF THEM
- [ ] PRACTICED BEING MORE PRESENT WITH OTHERS
- [ ] SHARED A STORY
- [ ] WROTE A PERSONAL NOTE OR TEXT

REFLECT

HOW I'D RATE MY FEELING OF CONNECTION TODAY:

| 1 | 2 | 3 | 4 | 5 | 6 | 7 | 8 | 9 | 10 |

LONELY / DISCONNECTED   HIGHLY CONNECTED

THE MOST MEANINGFUL INTERACTION I HAD TODAY AND HOW IT MADE ME FEEL:

_____
_____
_____
_____
_____
_____
_____
_____

CHALLENGES TO DEVELOPING DEEPER BONDS AND HOW I CAN OVERCOME THEM:

_____
_____
_____
_____

WAYS I'D LIKE TO CONNECT MORE:

_____
_____
_____
_____
_____

RECORD

DATE ___/___/___

MY GOALS FOR MEANINGFUL CONNECTIONS TODAY:

- [ ] _____
- [ ] _____
- [ ] _____

PEOPLE I'D LIKE TO CONNECT WITH:

WAYS TO STRENGTHEN MY RELATIONSHIPS:

WAYS I CONNECTED WITH OTHERS TODAY:

- [ ] CALLED A FRIEND
- [ ] ENCOURAGED SOMEONE
- [ ] ASKED FOR HELP OR ADVICE
- [ ] PLANNED ONE-ON-ONE TIME
- [ ] PRACTICED ACTIVE LISTENING
- [ ] EXPRESSED MY GRATITUDE TO SOMEONE ELSE
- [ ] SPENT QUALITY TIME WITH A FRIEND OR FAMILY MEMBER
- [ ] HELPED SOMEONE
- [ ] SHARED SOMETHING PERSONAL ABOUT MYSELF
- [ ] PRACTICED VULNERABILITY WITH A TRUSTED FRIEND
- [ ] SHARED A LAUGH
- [ ] TALKED TO SOMEONE NEW
- [ ] COMPLIMENTED SOMEONE
- [ ] COMPLETED A SHARED ACTIVITY
- [ ] NOTED SOMEONE ELSE'S MEANINGFUL DATE, EVENT, OR INTEREST I'D LIKE TO REMEMBER
- [ ] LET SOMEONE KNOW I WAS THINKING OF THEM
- [ ] PRACTICED BEING MORE PRESENT WITH OTHERS
- [ ] SHARED A STORY
- [ ] WROTE A PERSONAL NOTE OR TEXT

REFLECT

HOW I'D RATE MY FEELING OF CONNECTION TODAY:

| 1 | 2 | 3 | 4 | 5 | 6 | 7 | 8 | 9 | 10 |

LONELY / DISCONNECTED   HIGHLY CONNECTED

THE MOST MEANINGFUL INTERACTION I HAD TODAY AND HOW IT MADE ME FEEL:

___

CHALLENGES TO DEVELOPING DEEPER BONDS AND HOW I CAN OVERCOME THEM:

___

WAYS I'D LIKE TO CONNECT MORE:

___

RECORD

DATE ___/___/___

MY GOALS FOR MEANINGFUL CONNECTIONS TODAY:

- [ ] _____
- [ ] _____
- [ ] _____

PEOPLE I'D LIKE TO CONNECT WITH:
_____
_____

WAYS TO STRENGTHEN MY RELATIONSHIPS:
_____
_____

WAYS I CONNECTED WITH OTHERS TODAY:

- [ ] CALLED A FRIEND
- [ ] ENCOURAGED SOMEONE
- [ ] ASKED FOR HELP OR ADVICE
- [ ] PLANNED ONE-ON-ONE TIME
- [ ] PRACTICED ACTIVE LISTENING
- [ ] EXPRESSED MY GRATITUDE TO SOMEONE ELSE
- [ ] SPENT QUALITY TIME WITH A FRIEND OR FAMILY MEMBER
- [ ] HELPED SOMEONE
- [ ] SHARED SOMETHING PERSONAL ABOUT MYSELF
- [ ] PRACTICED VULNERABILITY WITH A TRUSTED FRIEND
- [ ] SHARED A LAUGH
- [ ] TALKED TO SOMEONE NEW
- [ ] COMPLIMENTED SOMEONE
- [ ] COMPLETED A SHARED ACTIVITY
- [ ] NOTED SOMEONE ELSE'S MEANINGFUL DATE, EVENT, OR INTEREST I'D LIKE TO REMEMBER
- [ ] LET SOMEONE KNOW I WAS THINKING OF THEM
- [ ] PRACTICED BEING MORE PRESENT WITH OTHERS
- [ ] SHARED A STORY
- [ ] WROTE A PERSONAL NOTE OR TEXT

REFLECT

HOW I'D RATE MY FEELING OF CONNECTION TODAY:

| 1 | 2 | 3 | 4 | 5 | 6 | 7 | 8 | 9 | 10 |

LONELY / DISCONNECTED   HIGHLY CONNECTED

THE MOST MEANINGFUL INTERACTION I HAD
TODAY AND HOW IT MADE ME FEEL:

_____
_____
_____
_____
_____
_____
_____
_____

CHALLENGES TO DEVELOPING DEEPER BONDS
AND HOW I CAN OVERCOME THEM:

_____
_____
_____
_____

WAYS I'D LIKE TO CONNECT MORE:

_____
_____
_____
_____
_____

RECORD

DATE ___/___/___

MY GOALS FOR MEANINGFUL CONNECTIONS TODAY:

- [ ] _____
- [ ] _____
- [ ] _____

PEOPLE I'D LIKE TO CONNECT WITH:

_____
_____

WAYS TO STRENGTHEN MY RELATIONSHIPS:

_____
_____

WAYS I CONNECTED WITH OTHERS TODAY:

- [ ] CALLED A FRIEND
- [ ] ENCOURAGED SOMEONE
- [ ] ASKED FOR HELP OR ADVICE
- [ ] PLANNED ONE-ON-ONE TIME
- [ ] PRACTICED ACTIVE LISTENING
- [ ] EXPRESSED MY GRATITUDE TO SOMEONE ELSE
- [ ] SPENT QUALITY TIME WITH A FRIEND OR FAMILY MEMBER
- [ ] HELPED SOMEONE
- [ ] SHARED SOMETHING PERSONAL ABOUT MYSELF
- [ ] PRACTICED VULNERABILITY WITH A TRUSTED FRIEND
- [ ] SHARED A LAUGH
- [ ] TALKED TO SOMEONE NEW
- [ ] COMPLIMENTED SOMEONE
- [ ] COMPLETED A SHARED ACTIVITY
- [ ] NOTED SOMEONE ELSE'S MEANINGFUL DATE, EVENT, OR INTEREST I'D LIKE TO REMEMBER
- [ ] LET SOMEONE KNOW I WAS THINKING OF THEM
- [ ] PRACTICED BEING MORE PRESENT WITH OTHERS
- [ ] SHARED A STORY
- [ ] WROTE A PERSONAL NOTE OR TEXT

REFLECT

HOW I'D RATE MY FEELING OF CONNECTION TODAY:

| 1 | 2 | 3 | 4 | 5 | 6 | 7 | 8 | 9 | 10 |

LONELY / DISCONNECTED   HIGHLY CONNECTED

THE MOST MEANINGFUL INTERACTION I HAD TODAY AND HOW IT MADE ME FEEL:

___

CHALLENGES TO DEVELOPING DEEPER BONDS AND HOW I CAN OVERCOME THEM:

___

WAYS I'D LIKE TO CONNECT MORE:

___

RECORD

DATE ___/___/___

MY GOALS FOR MEANINGFUL CONNECTIONS TODAY:

- [ ] _____
- [ ] _____
- [ ] _____

PEOPLE I'D LIKE TO CONNECT WITH:
_____
_____

WAYS TO STRENGTHEN MY RELATIONSHIPS:
_____
_____

WAYS I CONNECTED WITH OTHERS TODAY:

- [ ] CALLED A FRIEND
- [ ] ENCOURAGED SOMEONE
- [ ] ASKED FOR HELP OR ADVICE
- [ ] PLANNED ONE-ON-ONE TIME
- [ ] PRACTICED ACTIVE LISTENING
- [ ] EXPRESSED MY GRATITUDE TO SOMEONE ELSE
- [ ] SPENT QUALITY TIME WITH A FRIEND OR FAMILY MEMBER
- [ ] HELPED SOMEONE
- [ ] SHARED SOMETHING PERSONAL ABOUT MYSELF
- [ ] PRACTICED VULNERABILITY WITH A TRUSTED FRIEND
- [ ] SHARED A LAUGH
- [ ] TALKED TO SOMEONE NEW
- [ ] COMPLIMENTED SOMEONE
- [ ] COMPLETED A SHARED ACTIVITY
- [ ] NOTED SOMEONE ELSE'S MEANINGFUL DATE, EVENT, OR INTEREST I'D LIKE TO REMEMBER
- [ ] LET SOMEONE KNOW I WAS THINKING OF THEM
- [ ] PRACTICED BEING MORE PRESENT WITH OTHERS
- [ ] SHARED A STORY
- [ ] WROTE A PERSONAL NOTE OR TEXT

REFLECT

HOW I'D RATE MY FEELING OF CONNECTION TODAY:

| 1 | 2 | 3 | 4 | 5 | 6 | 7 | 8 | 9 | 10 |

LONELY / DISCONNECTED   HIGHLY CONNECTED

THE MOST MEANINGFUL INTERACTION I HAD TODAY AND HOW IT MADE ME FEEL:

_____
_____
_____
_____
_____
_____
_____
_____

CHALLENGES TO DEVELOPING DEEPER BONDS AND HOW I CAN OVERCOME THEM:

_____
_____
_____

WAYS I'D LIKE TO CONNECT MORE:

_____
_____
_____
_____
_____

RECORD

DATE ___/___/___

MY GOALS FOR MEANINGFUL CONNECTIONS TODAY:

- ☐ _____
- ☐ _____
- ☐ _____

PEOPLE I'D LIKE TO CONNECT WITH:

_____
_____

WAYS TO STRENGTHEN MY RELATIONSHIPS:

_____
_____

WAYS I CONNECTED WITH OTHERS TODAY:

- ☐ CALLED A FRIEND
- ☐ ENCOURAGED SOMEONE
- ☐ ASKED FOR HELP OR ADVICE
- ☐ PLANNED ONE-ON-ONE TIME
- ☐ PRACTICED ACTIVE LISTENING
- ☐ EXPRESSED MY GRATITUDE TO SOMEONE ELSE
- ☐ SPENT QUALITY TIME WITH A FRIEND OR FAMILY MEMBER
- ☐ HELPED SOMEONE
- ☐ SHARED SOMETHING PERSONAL ABOUT MYSELF
- ☐ PRACTICED VULNERABILITY WITH A TRUSTED FRIEND
- ☐ SHARED A LAUGH
- ☐ TALKED TO SOMEONE NEW
- ☐ COMPLIMENTED SOMEONE
- ☐ COMPLETED A SHARED ACTIVITY
- ☐ NOTED SOMEONE ELSE'S MEANINGFUL DATE, EVENT, OR INTEREST I'D LIKE TO REMEMBER
- ☐ LET SOMEONE KNOW I WAS THINKING OF THEM
- ☐ PRACTICED BEING MORE PRESENT WITH OTHERS
- ☐ SHARED A STORY
- ☐ WROTE A PERSONAL NOTE OR TEXT

REFLECT

HOW I'D RATE MY FEELING OF CONNECTION TODAY:

| 1 | 2 | 3 | 4 | 5 | 6 | 7 | 8 | 9 | 10 |

LONELY / DISCONNECTED   HIGHLY CONNECTED

THE MOST MEANINGFUL INTERACTION I HAD TODAY AND HOW IT MADE ME FEEL:

_____
_____
_____
_____
_____
_____
_____
_____

CHALLENGES TO DEVELOPING DEEPER BONDS AND HOW I CAN OVERCOME THEM:

_____
_____
_____
_____

WAYS I'D LIKE TO CONNECT MORE:

_____
_____
_____
_____

RECORD

DATE ___/___/___

MY GOALS FOR MEANINGFUL CONNECTIONS TODAY:
- [ ] _____
- [ ] _____
- [ ] _____

PEOPLE I'D LIKE TO CONNECT WITH:
_____
_____

WAYS TO STRENGTHEN MY RELATIONSHIPS:
_____
_____

WAYS I CONNECTED WITH OTHERS TODAY:

- [ ] CALLED A FRIEND
- [ ] ENCOURAGED SOMEONE
- [ ] ASKED FOR HELP OR ADVICE
- [ ] PLANNED ONE-ON-ONE TIME
- [ ] PRACTICED ACTIVE LISTENING
- [ ] EXPRESSED MY GRATITUDE TO SOMEONE ELSE
- [ ] SPENT QUALITY TIME WITH A FRIEND OR FAMILY MEMBER
- [ ] HELPED SOMEONE
- [ ] SHARED SOMETHING PERSONAL ABOUT MYSELF
- [ ] PRACTICED VULNERABILITY WITH A TRUSTED FRIEND
- [ ] SHARED A LAUGH
- [ ] TALKED TO SOMEONE NEW
- [ ] COMPLIMENTED SOMEONE
- [ ] COMPLETED A SHARED ACTIVITY
- [ ] NOTED SOMEONE ELSE'S MEANINGFUL DATE, EVENT, OR INTEREST I'D LIKE TO REMEMBER
- [ ] LET SOMEONE KNOW I WAS THINKING OF THEM
- [ ] PRACTICED BEING MORE PRESENT WITH OTHERS
- [ ] SHARED A STORY
- [ ] WROTE A PERSONAL NOTE OR TEXT

REFLECT

HOW I'D RATE MY FEELING OF CONNECTION TODAY:

| 1 | 2 | 3 | 4 | 5 | 6 | 7 | 8 | 9 | 10 |

LONELY / DISCONNECTED   HIGHLY CONNECTED

THE MOST MEANINGFUL INTERACTION I HAD TODAY AND HOW IT MADE ME FEEL:

_____
_____
_____
_____
_____
_____

CHALLENGES TO DEVELOPING DEEPER BONDS AND HOW I CAN OVERCOME THEM:

_____
_____
_____
_____

WAYS I'D LIKE TO CONNECT MORE:

_____
_____
_____
_____

RECORD

DATE ___/___/___

MY GOALS FOR MEANINGFUL CONNECTIONS TODAY:

- ☐ _____
- ☐ _____
- ☐ _____

PEOPLE I'D LIKE TO CONNECT WITH:

_____
_____

WAYS TO STRENGTHEN MY RELATIONSHIPS:

_____
_____

WAYS I CONNECTED WITH OTHERS TODAY:

- ☐ CALLED A FRIEND
- ☐ ENCOURAGED SOMEONE
- ☐ ASKED FOR HELP OR ADVICE
- ☐ PLANNED ONE-ON-ONE TIME
- ☐ PRACTICED ACTIVE LISTENING
- ☐ EXPRESSED MY GRATITUDE TO SOMEONE ELSE
- ☐ SPENT QUALITY TIME WITH A FRIEND OR FAMILY MEMBER
- ☐ HELPED SOMEONE
- ☐ SHARED SOMETHING PERSONAL ABOUT MYSELF
- ☐ PRACTICED VULNERABILITY WITH A TRUSTED FRIEND
- ☐ SHARED A LAUGH
- ☐ TALKED TO SOMEONE NEW
- ☐ COMPLIMENTED SOMEONE
- ☐ COMPLETED A SHARED ACTIVITY
- ☐ NOTED SOMEONE ELSE'S MEANINGFUL DATE, EVENT, OR INTEREST I'D LIKE TO REMEMBER
- ☐ LET SOMEONE KNOW I WAS THINKING OF THEM
- ☐ PRACTICED BEING MORE PRESENT WITH OTHERS
- ☐ SHARED A STORY
- ☐ WROTE A PERSONAL NOTE OR TEXT

REFLECT

HOW I'D RATE MY FEELING OF CONNECTION TODAY:

| 1 | 2 | 3 | 4 | 5 | 6 | 7 | 8 | 9 | 10 |

LONELY / DISCONNECTED   HIGHLY CONNECTED

THE MOST MEANINGFUL INTERACTION I HAD TODAY AND HOW IT MADE ME FEEL:

_____
_____
_____
_____
_____
_____
_____
_____

CHALLENGES TO DEVELOPING DEEPER BONDS AND HOW I CAN OVERCOME THEM:

_____
_____
_____
_____

WAYS I'D LIKE TO CONNECT MORE:

_____
_____
_____
_____
_____

RECORD

DATE ___/___/___

MY GOALS FOR MEANINGFUL CONNECTIONS TODAY:
- [ ] _____
- [ ] _____
- [ ] _____

PEOPLE I'D LIKE TO CONNECT WITH:
_____
_____

WAYS TO STRENGTHEN MY RELATIONSHIPS:
_____
_____

WAYS I CONNECTED WITH OTHERS TODAY:

- [ ] CALLED A FRIEND
- [ ] ENCOURAGED SOMEONE
- [ ] ASKED FOR HELP OR ADVICE
- [ ] PLANNED ONE-ON-ONE TIME
- [ ] PRACTICED ACTIVE LISTENING
- [ ] EXPRESSED MY GRATITUDE TO SOMEONE ELSE
- [ ] SPENT QUALITY TIME WITH A FRIEND OR FAMILY MEMBER
- [ ] HELPED SOMEONE
- [ ] SHARED SOMETHING PERSONAL ABOUT MYSELF
- [ ] PRACTICED VULNERABILITY WITH A TRUSTED FRIEND
- [ ] SHARED A LAUGH
- [ ] TALKED TO SOMEONE NEW
- [ ] COMPLIMENTED SOMEONE
- [ ] COMPLETED A SHARED ACTIVITY
- [ ] NOTED SOMEONE ELSE'S MEANINGFUL DATE, EVENT, OR INTEREST I'D LIKE TO REMEMBER
- [ ] LET SOMEONE KNOW I WAS THINKING OF THEM
- [ ] PRACTICED BEING MORE PRESENT WITH OTHERS
- [ ] SHARED A STORY
- [ ] WROTE A PERSONAL NOTE OR TEXT

REFLECT

HOW I'D RATE MY FEELING OF CONNECTION TODAY:

1 2 3 4 5 6 7 8 9 10

LONELY / DISCONNECTED   HIGHLY CONNECTED

THE MOST MEANINGFUL INTERACTION I HAD TODAY AND HOW IT MADE ME FEEL:

_____
_____
_____
_____
_____
_____
_____

CHALLENGES TO DEVELOPING DEEPER BONDS AND HOW I CAN OVERCOME THEM:

_____
_____
_____
_____

WAYS I'D LIKE TO CONNECT MORE:

_____
_____
_____
_____

RECORD

DATE ___/___/___

MY GOALS FOR MEANINGFUL CONNECTIONS TODAY:
- ☐ _____
- ☐ _____
- ☐ _____

PEOPLE I'D LIKE TO CONNECT WITH:
_____
_____

WAYS TO STRENGTHEN MY RELATIONSHIPS:
_____
_____

WAYS I CONNECTED WITH OTHERS TODAY:

- ☐ CALLED A FRIEND
- ☐ ENCOURAGED SOMEONE
- ☐ ASKED FOR HELP OR ADVICE
- ☐ PLANNED ONE-ON-ONE TIME
- ☐ PRACTICED ACTIVE LISTENING
- ☐ EXPRESSED MY GRATITUDE TO SOMEONE ELSE
- ☐ SPENT QUALITY TIME WITH A FRIEND OR FAMILY MEMBER
- ☐ HELPED SOMEONE
- ☐ SHARED SOMETHING PERSONAL ABOUT MYSELF
- ☐ PRACTICED VULNERABILITY WITH A TRUSTED FRIEND
- ☐ SHARED A LAUGH
- ☐ TALKED TO SOMEONE NEW
- ☐ COMPLIMENTED SOMEONE
- ☐ COMPLETED A SHARED ACTIVITY
- ☐ NOTED SOMEONE ELSE'S MEANINGFUL DATE, EVENT, OR INTEREST I'D LIKE TO REMEMBER
- ☐ LET SOMEONE KNOW I WAS THINKING OF THEM
- ☐ PRACTICED BEING MORE PRESENT WITH OTHERS
- ☐ SHARED A STORY
- ☐ WROTE A PERSONAL NOTE OR TEXT

REFLECT

HOW I'D RATE MY FEELING OF CONNECTION TODAY:

| 1 | 2 | 3 | 4 | 5 | 6 | 7 | 8 | 9 | 10 |

LONELY / DISCONNECTED HIGHLY CONNECTED

THE MOST MEANINGFUL INTERACTION I HAD TODAY AND HOW IT MADE ME FEEL:

CHALLENGES TO DEVELOPING DEEPER BONDS AND HOW I CAN OVERCOME THEM:

WAYS I'D LIKE TO CONNECT MORE:

RECORD

DATE ___/___/___

MY GOALS FOR MEANINGFUL CONNECTIONS TODAY:

- [ ] _____
- [ ] _____
- [ ] _____

PEOPLE I'D LIKE TO CONNECT WITH:

_____
_____

WAYS TO STRENGTHEN MY RELATIONSHIPS:

_____
_____

WAYS I CONNECTED WITH OTHERS TODAY:

- [ ] CALLED A FRIEND
- [ ] ENCOURAGED SOMEONE
- [ ] ASKED FOR HELP OR ADVICE
- [ ] PLANNED ONE-ON-ONE TIME
- [ ] PRACTICED ACTIVE LISTENING
- [ ] EXPRESSED MY GRATITUDE TO SOMEONE ELSE
- [ ] SPENT QUALITY TIME WITH A FRIEND OR FAMILY MEMBER
- [ ] HELPED SOMEONE
- [ ] SHARED SOMETHING PERSONAL ABOUT MYSELF
- [ ] PRACTICED VULNERABILITY WITH A TRUSTED FRIEND
- [ ] SHARED A LAUGH
- [ ] TALKED TO SOMEONE NEW
- [ ] COMPLIMENTED SOMEONE
- [ ] COMPLETED A SHARED ACTIVITY
- [ ] NOTED SOMEONE ELSE'S MEANINGFUL DATE, EVENT, OR INTEREST I'D LIKE TO REMEMBER
- [ ] LET SOMEONE KNOW I WAS THINKING OF THEM
- [ ] PRACTICED BEING MORE PRESENT WITH OTHERS
- [ ] SHARED A STORY
- [ ] WROTE A PERSONAL NOTE OR TEXT

REFLECT

HOW I'D RATE MY FEELING OF CONNECTION TODAY:

| 1 | 2 | 3 | 4 | 5 | 6 | 7 | 8 | 9 | 10 |

LONELY / DISCONNECTED   HIGHLY CONNECTED

THE MOST MEANINGFUL INTERACTION I HAD TODAY AND HOW IT MADE ME FEEL:

_____
_____
_____
_____
_____
_____
_____
_____
_____

CHALLENGES TO DEVELOPING DEEPER BONDS AND HOW I CAN OVERCOME THEM:

_____
_____
_____
_____

WAYS I'D LIKE TO CONNECT MORE:

_____
_____
_____
_____
_____

RECORD

DATE ___/___/___

MY GOALS FOR MEANINGFUL CONNECTIONS TODAY:

- [ ] _____
- [ ] _____
- [ ] _____

PEOPLE I'D LIKE TO CONNECT WITH:
_____
_____

WAYS TO STRENGTHEN MY RELATIONSHIPS:
_____
_____

WAYS I CONNECTED WITH OTHERS TODAY:

- [ ] CALLED A FRIEND
- [ ] ENCOURAGED SOMEONE
- [ ] ASKED FOR HELP OR ADVICE
- [ ] PLANNED ONE-ON-ONE TIME
- [ ] PRACTICED ACTIVE LISTENING
- [ ] EXPRESSED MY GRATITUDE TO SOMEONE ELSE
- [ ] SPENT QUALITY TIME WITH A FRIEND OR FAMILY MEMBER
- [ ] HELPED SOMEONE
- [ ] SHARED SOMETHING PERSONAL ABOUT MYSELF
- [ ] PRACTICED VULNERABILITY WITH A TRUSTED FRIEND
- [ ] SHARED A LAUGH
- [ ] TALKED TO SOMEONE NEW
- [ ] COMPLIMENTED SOMEONE
- [ ] COMPLETED A SHARED ACTIVITY
- [ ] NOTED SOMEONE ELSE'S MEANINGFUL DATE, EVENT, OR INTEREST I'D LIKE TO REMEMBER
- [ ] LET SOMEONE KNOW I WAS THINKING OF THEM
- [ ] PRACTICED BEING MORE PRESENT WITH OTHERS
- [ ] SHARED A STORY
- [ ] WROTE A PERSONAL NOTE OR TEXT

REFLECT

HOW I'D RATE MY FEELING OF CONNECTION TODAY:

| 1 | 2 | 3 | 4 | 5 | 6 | 7 | 8 | 9 | 10 |

LONELY / DISCONNECTED   HIGHLY CONNECTED

THE MOST MEANINGFUL INTERACTION I HAD TODAY AND HOW IT MADE ME FEEL:

_____
_____
_____
_____
_____
_____
_____
_____

CHALLENGES TO DEVELOPING DEEPER BONDS AND HOW I CAN OVERCOME THEM:

_____
_____
_____
_____

WAYS I'D LIKE TO CONNECT MORE:

_____
_____
_____
_____
_____

RECORD

DATE ___/___/___

MY GOALS FOR MEANINGFUL CONNECTIONS TODAY:

- ☐ _____
- ☐ _____
- ☐ _____

PEOPLE I'D LIKE TO CONNECT WITH:

_____
_____

WAYS TO STRENGTHEN MY RELATIONSHIPS:

_____
_____

WAYS I CONNECTED WITH OTHERS TODAY:

- ☐ CALLED A FRIEND
- ☐ ENCOURAGED SOMEONE
- ☐ ASKED FOR HELP OR ADVICE
- ☐ PLANNED ONE-ON-ONE TIME
- ☐ PRACTICED ACTIVE LISTENING
- ☐ EXPRESSED MY GRATITUDE TO SOMEONE ELSE
- ☐ SPENT QUALITY TIME WITH A FRIEND OR FAMILY MEMBER
- ☐ HELPED SOMEONE
- ☐ SHARED SOMETHING PERSONAL ABOUT MYSELF
- ☐ PRACTICED VULNERABILITY WITH A TRUSTED FRIEND
- ☐ SHARED A LAUGH
- ☐ TALKED TO SOMEONE NEW
- ☐ COMPLIMENTED SOMEONE
- ☐ COMPLETED A SHARED ACTIVITY
- ☐ NOTED SOMEONE ELSE'S MEANINGFUL DATE, EVENT, OR INTEREST I'D LIKE TO REMEMBER
- ☐ LET SOMEONE KNOW I WAS THINKING OF THEM
- ☐ PRACTICED BEING MORE PRESENT WITH OTHERS
- ☐ SHARED A STORY
- ☐ WROTE A PERSONAL NOTE OR TEXT

REFLECT

HOW I'D RATE MY FEELING OF CONNECTION TODAY:

| 1 | 2 | 3 | 4 | 5 | 6 | 7 | 8 | 9 | 10 |

LONELY / DISCONNECTED　　　　　　　　　　　　　　　　　HIGHLY CONNECTED

THE MOST MEANINGFUL INTERACTION I HAD TODAY AND HOW IT MADE ME FEEL:

_____
_____
_____
_____
_____
_____
_____
_____

CHALLENGES TO DEVELOPING DEEPER BONDS AND HOW I CAN OVERCOME THEM:

_____
_____
_____
_____

WAYS I'D LIKE TO CONNECT MORE:

_____
_____
_____
_____
_____

RECORD

DATE ___/___/___

MY GOALS FOR MEANINGFUL CONNECTIONS TODAY:

- ☐ _____
- ☐ _____
- ☐ _____

PEOPLE I'D LIKE TO CONNECT WITH:

_____
_____

WAYS TO STRENGTHEN MY RELATIONSHIPS:

_____
_____

WAYS I CONNECTED WITH OTHERS TODAY:

- ☐ CALLED A FRIEND
- ☐ ENCOURAGED SOMEONE
- ☐ ASKED FOR HELP OR ADVICE
- ☐ PLANNED ONE-ON-ONE TIME
- ☐ PRACTICED ACTIVE LISTENING
- ☐ EXPRESSED MY GRATITUDE TO SOMEONE ELSE
- ☐ SPENT QUALITY TIME WITH A FRIEND OR FAMILY MEMBER
- ☐ HELPED SOMEONE
- ☐ SHARED SOMETHING PERSONAL ABOUT MYSELF
- ☐ PRACTICED VULNERABILITY WITH A TRUSTED FRIEND
- ☐ SHARED A LAUGH
- ☐ TALKED TO SOMEONE NEW
- ☐ COMPLIMENTED SOMEONE
- ☐ COMPLETED A SHARED ACTIVITY
- ☐ NOTED SOMEONE ELSE'S MEANINGFUL DATE, EVENT, OR INTEREST I'D LIKE TO REMEMBER
- ☐ LET SOMEONE KNOW I WAS THINKING OF THEM
- ☐ PRACTICED BEING MORE PRESENT WITH OTHERS
- ☐ SHARED A STORY
- ☐ WROTE A PERSONAL NOTE OR TEXT

REFLECT

HOW I'D RATE MY FEELING OF CONNECTION TODAY:

| 1 | 2 | 3 | 4 | 5 | 6 | 7 | 8 | 9 | 10 |

LONELY / DISCONNECTED   HIGHLY CONNECTED

THE MOST MEANINGFUL INTERACTION I HAD TODAY AND HOW IT MADE ME FEEL:

_____
_____
_____
_____
_____
_____
_____
_____

CHALLENGES TO DEVELOPING DEEPER BONDS AND HOW I CAN OVERCOME THEM:

_____
_____
_____
_____

WAYS I'D LIKE TO CONNECT MORE:

_____
_____
_____
_____
_____

RECORD

DATE ___/___/___

MY GOALS FOR MEANINGFUL CONNECTIONS TODAY:

- [ ] _____
- [ ] _____
- [ ] _____

PEOPLE I'D LIKE TO CONNECT WITH:

_____
_____

WAYS TO STRENGTHEN MY RELATIONSHIPS:

_____
_____

WAYS I CONNECTED WITH OTHERS TODAY:

- [ ] CALLED A FRIEND
- [ ] ENCOURAGED SOMEONE
- [ ] ASKED FOR HELP OR ADVICE
- [ ] PLANNED ONE-ON-ONE TIME
- [ ] PRACTICED ACTIVE LISTENING
- [ ] EXPRESSED MY GRATITUDE TO SOMEONE ELSE
- [ ] SPENT QUALITY TIME WITH A FRIEND OR FAMILY MEMBER
- [ ] HELPED SOMEONE
- [ ] SHARED SOMETHING PERSONAL ABOUT MYSELF
- [ ] PRACTICED VULNERABILITY WITH A TRUSTED FRIEND
- [ ] SHARED A LAUGH
- [ ] TALKED TO SOMEONE NEW
- [ ] COMPLIMENTED SOMEONE
- [ ] COMPLETED A SHARED ACTIVITY
- [ ] NOTED SOMEONE ELSE'S MEANINGFUL DATE, EVENT, OR INTEREST I'D LIKE TO REMEMBER
- [ ] LET SOMEONE KNOW I WAS THINKING OF THEM
- [ ] PRACTICED BEING MORE PRESENT WITH OTHERS
- [ ] SHARED A STORY
- [ ] WROTE A PERSONAL NOTE OR TEXT

REFLECT

HOW I'D RATE MY FEELING OF CONNECTION TODAY:

| 1 | 2 | 3 | 4 | 5 | 6 | 7 | 8 | 9 | 10 |

LONELY / DISCONNECTED   HIGHLY CONNECTED

THE MOST MEANINGFUL INTERACTION I HAD TODAY AND HOW IT MADE ME FEEL:

_____
_____
_____
_____
_____
_____
_____
_____

CHALLENGES TO DEVELOPING DEEPER BONDS AND HOW I CAN OVERCOME THEM:

_____
_____
_____
_____

WAYS I'D LIKE TO CONNECT MORE:

_____
_____
_____
_____

RECORD

DATE ___ / ___ / ___

MY GOALS FOR MEANINGFUL CONNECTIONS TODAY:

- ☐ _____
- ☐ _____
- ☐ _____

PEOPLE I'D LIKE TO CONNECT WITH:

_____
_____

WAYS TO STRENGTHEN MY RELATIONSHIPS:

_____
_____

WAYS I CONNECTED WITH OTHERS TODAY:

- ☐ CALLED A FRIEND
- ☐ ENCOURAGED SOMEONE
- ☐ ASKED FOR HELP OR ADVICE
- ☐ PLANNED ONE-ON-ONE TIME
- ☐ PRACTICED ACTIVE LISTENING
- ☐ EXPRESSED MY GRATITUDE TO SOMEONE ELSE
- ☐ SPENT QUALITY TIME WITH A FRIEND OR FAMILY MEMBER
- ☐ HELPED SOMEONE
- ☐ SHARED SOMETHING PERSONAL ABOUT MYSELF
- ☐ PRACTICED VULNERABILITY WITH A TRUSTED FRIEND
- ☐ SHARED A LAUGH
- ☐ TALKED TO SOMEONE NEW
- ☐ COMPLIMENTED SOMEONE
- ☐ COMPLETED A SHARED ACTIVITY
- ☐ NOTED SOMEONE ELSE'S MEANINGFUL DATE, EVENT, OR INTEREST I'D LIKE TO REMEMBER
- ☐ LET SOMEONE KNOW I WAS THINKING OF THEM
- ☐ PRACTICED BEING MORE PRESENT WITH OTHERS
- ☐ SHARED A STORY
- ☐ WROTE A PERSONAL NOTE OR TEXT

REFLECT

HOW I'D RATE MY FEELING OF CONNECTION TODAY:

| 1 | 2 | 3 | 4 | 5 | 6 | 7 | 8 | 9 | 10 |

LONELY / DISCONNECTED   HIGHLY CONNECTED

THE MOST MEANINGFUL INTERACTION I HAD TODAY AND HOW IT MADE ME FEEL:

_____
_____
_____
_____
_____
_____
_____
_____
_____

CHALLENGES TO DEVELOPING DEEPER BONDS AND HOW I CAN OVERCOME THEM:

_____
_____
_____
_____

WAYS I'D LIKE TO CONNECT MORE:

_____
_____
_____
_____

RECORD

DATE ___/___/___

MY GOALS FOR MEANINGFUL CONNECTIONS TODAY:

- ☐ _____
- ☐ _____
- ☐ _____

PEOPLE I'D LIKE TO CONNECT WITH:

_____
_____

WAYS TO STRENGTHEN MY RELATIONSHIPS:

_____
_____

WAYS I CONNECTED WITH OTHERS TODAY:

- ☐ CALLED A FRIEND
- ☐ ENCOURAGED SOMEONE
- ☐ ASKED FOR HELP OR ADVICE
- ☐ PLANNED ONE-ON-ONE TIME
- ☐ PRACTICED ACTIVE LISTENING
- ☐ EXPRESSED MY GRATITUDE TO SOMEONE ELSE
- ☐ SPENT QUALITY TIME WITH A FRIEND OR FAMILY MEMBER
- ☐ HELPED SOMEONE
- ☐ SHARED SOMETHING PERSONAL ABOUT MYSELF
- ☐ PRACTICED VULNERABILITY WITH A TRUSTED FRIEND
- ☐ SHARED A LAUGH
- ☐ TALKED TO SOMEONE NEW
- ☐ COMPLIMENTED SOMEONE
- ☐ COMPLETED A SHARED ACTIVITY
- ☐ NOTED SOMEONE ELSE'S MEANINGFUL DATE, EVENT, OR INTEREST I'D LIKE TO REMEMBER
- ☐ LET SOMEONE KNOW I WAS THINKING OF THEM
- ☐ PRACTICED BEING MORE PRESENT WITH OTHERS
- ☐ SHARED A STORY
- ☐ WROTE A PERSONAL NOTE OR TEXT

REFLECT

HOW I'D RATE MY FEELING OF CONNECTION TODAY:

| 1 | 2 | 3 | 4 | 5 | 6 | 7 | 8 | 9 | 10 |

LONELY / DISCONNECTEDHIGHLY CONNECTED

THE MOST MEANINGFUL INTERACTION I HAD TODAY AND HOW IT MADE ME FEEL:

_____
_____
_____
_____
_____
_____
_____
_____

CHALLENGES TO DEVELOPING DEEPER BONDS AND HOW I CAN OVERCOME THEM:

_____
_____
_____
_____

WAYS I'D LIKE TO CONNECT MORE:

_____
_____
_____
_____
_____

RECORD

DATE ___/___/___

MY GOALS FOR MEANINGFUL CONNECTIONS TODAY:

- [ ] _____
- [ ] _____
- [ ] _____

PEOPLE I'D LIKE TO CONNECT WITH:

_____
_____

WAYS TO STRENGTHEN MY RELATIONSHIPS:

_____
_____

WAYS I CONNECTED WITH OTHERS TODAY:

- [ ] CALLED A FRIEND
- [ ] ENCOURAGED SOMEONE
- [ ] ASKED FOR HELP OR ADVICE
- [ ] PLANNED ONE-ON-ONE TIME
- [ ] PRACTICED ACTIVE LISTENING
- [ ] EXPRESSED MY GRATITUDE TO SOMEONE ELSE
- [ ] SPENT QUALITY TIME WITH A FRIEND OR FAMILY MEMBER
- [ ] HELPED SOMEONE
- [ ] SHARED SOMETHING PERSONAL ABOUT MYSELF
- [ ] PRACTICED VULNERABILITY WITH A TRUSTED FRIEND
- [ ] SHARED A LAUGH
- [ ] TALKED TO SOMEONE NEW
- [ ] COMPLIMENTED SOMEONE
- [ ] COMPLETED A SHARED ACTIVITY
- [ ] NOTED SOMEONE ELSE'S MEANINGFUL DATE, EVENT, OR INTEREST I'D LIKE TO REMEMBER
- [ ] LET SOMEONE KNOW I WAS THINKING OF THEM
- [ ] PRACTICED BEING MORE PRESENT WITH OTHERS
- [ ] SHARED A STORY
- [ ] WROTE A PERSONAL NOTE OR TEXT

REFLECT

HOW I'D RATE MY FEELING OF CONNECTION TODAY:

| 1 | 2 | 3 | 4 | 5 | 6 | 7 | 8 | 9 | 10 |

LONELY / DISCONNECTED HIGHLY CONNECTED

THE MOST MEANINGFUL INTERACTION I HAD TODAY AND HOW IT MADE ME FEEL:

CHALLENGES TO DEVELOPING DEEPER BONDS AND HOW I CAN OVERCOME THEM:

WAYS I'D LIKE TO CONNECT MORE:

RECORD

DATE ___/___/___

MY GOALS FOR MEANINGFUL CONNECTIONS TODAY:

- [ ] _____
- [ ] _____
- [ ] _____

PEOPLE I'D LIKE TO CONNECT WITH:

_____
_____

WAYS TO STRENGTHEN MY RELATIONSHIPS:

_____
_____

WAYS I CONNECTED WITH OTHERS TODAY:

- [ ] CALLED A FRIEND
- [ ] ENCOURAGED SOMEONE
- [ ] ASKED FOR HELP OR ADVICE
- [ ] PLANNED ONE-ON-ONE TIME
- [ ] PRACTICED ACTIVE LISTENING
- [ ] EXPRESSED MY GRATITUDE TO SOMEONE ELSE
- [ ] SPENT QUALITY TIME WITH A FRIEND OR FAMILY MEMBER
- [ ] HELPED SOMEONE
- [ ] SHARED SOMETHING PERSONAL ABOUT MYSELF
- [ ] PRACTICED VULNERABILITY WITH A TRUSTED FRIEND
- [ ] SHARED A LAUGH
- [ ] TALKED TO SOMEONE NEW
- [ ] COMPLIMENTED SOMEONE
- [ ] COMPLETED A SHARED ACTIVITY
- [ ] NOTED SOMEONE ELSE'S MEANINGFUL DATE, EVENT, OR INTEREST I'D LIKE TO REMEMBER
- [ ] LET SOMEONE KNOW I WAS THINKING OF THEM
- [ ] PRACTICED BEING MORE PRESENT WITH OTHERS
- [ ] SHARED A STORY
- [ ] WROTE A PERSONAL NOTE OR TEXT

REFLECT

HOW I'D RATE MY FEELING OF CONNECTION TODAY:

| 1 | 2 | 3 | 4 | 5 | 6 | 7 | 8 | 9 | 10 |

LONELY / DISCONNECTED   HIGHLY CONNECTED

THE MOST MEANINGFUL INTERACTION I HAD TODAY AND HOW IT MADE ME FEEL:

_____
_____
_____
_____
_____
_____
_____
_____

CHALLENGES TO DEVELOPING DEEPER BONDS AND HOW I CAN OVERCOME THEM:

_____
_____
_____
_____

WAYS I'D LIKE TO CONNECT MORE:

_____
_____
_____
_____
_____

RECORD

DATE ___/___/___

MY GOALS FOR MEANINGFUL CONNECTIONS TODAY:
- ☐ _____
- ☐ _____
- ☐ _____

PEOPLE I'D LIKE TO CONNECT WITH:
_____
_____

WAYS TO STRENGTHEN MY RELATIONSHIPS:
_____
_____

WAYS I CONNECTED WITH OTHERS TODAY:

- ☐ CALLED A FRIEND
- ☐ ENCOURAGED SOMEONE
- ☐ ASKED FOR HELP OR ADVICE
- ☐ PLANNED ONE-ON-ONE TIME
- ☐ PRACTICED ACTIVE LISTENING
- ☐ EXPRESSED MY GRATITUDE TO SOMEONE ELSE
- ☐ SPENT QUALITY TIME WITH A FRIEND OR FAMILY MEMBER
- ☐ HELPED SOMEONE
- ☐ SHARED SOMETHING PERSONAL ABOUT MYSELF
- ☐ PRACTICED VULNERABILITY WITH A TRUSTED FRIEND
- ☐ SHARED A LAUGH
- ☐ TALKED TO SOMEONE NEW
- ☐ COMPLIMENTED SOMEONE
- ☐ COMPLETED A SHARED ACTIVITY
- ☐ NOTED SOMEONE ELSE'S MEANINGFUL DATE, EVENT, OR INTEREST I'D LIKE TO REMEMBER
- ☐ LET SOMEONE KNOW I WAS THINKING OF THEM
- ☐ PRACTICED BEING MORE PRESENT WITH OTHERS
- ☐ SHARED A STORY
- ☐ WROTE A PERSONAL NOTE OR TEXT

REFLECT

HOW I'D RATE MY FEELING OF CONNECTION TODAY:

| 1 | 2 | 3 | 4 | 5 | 6 | 7 | 8 | 9 | 10 |

LONELY / DISCONNECTED — HIGHLY CONNECTED

THE MOST MEANINGFUL INTERACTION
I HAD TODAY AND HOW IT MADE ME FEEL:

_____
_____
_____
_____
_____
_____
_____
_____
_____

CHALLENGES TO DEVELOPING DEEPER BONDS
AND HOW I CAN OVERCOME THEM:

_____
_____
_____

WAYS I'D LIKE TO CONNECT MORE:

_____
_____
_____
_____

RECORD

DATE ___/___/___

MY GOALS FOR MEANINGFUL CONNECTIONS TODAY:

- [ ] _____
- [ ] _____
- [ ] _____

PEOPLE I'D LIKE TO CONNECT WITH:

_____
_____

WAYS TO STRENGTHEN MY RELATIONSHIPS:

_____
_____

WAYS I CONNECTED WITH OTHERS TODAY:

- [ ] CALLED A FRIEND
- [ ] ENCOURAGED SOMEONE
- [ ] ASKED FOR HELP OR ADVICE
- [ ] PLANNED ONE-ON-ONE TIME
- [ ] PRACTICED ACTIVE LISTENING
- [ ] EXPRESSED MY GRATITUDE TO SOMEONE ELSE
- [ ] SPENT QUALITY TIME WITH A FRIEND OR FAMILY MEMBER
- [ ] HELPED SOMEONE
- [ ] SHARED SOMETHING PERSONAL ABOUT MYSELF
- [ ] PRACTICED VULNERABILITY WITH A TRUSTED FRIEND
- [ ] SHARED A LAUGH
- [ ] TALKED TO SOMEONE NEW
- [ ] COMPLIMENTED SOMEONE
- [ ] COMPLETED A SHARED ACTIVITY
- [ ] NOTED SOMEONE ELSE'S MEANINGFUL DATE, EVENT, OR INTEREST I'D LIKE TO REMEMBER
- [ ] LET SOMEONE KNOW I WAS THINKING OF THEM
- [ ] PRACTICED BEING MORE PRESENT WITH OTHERS
- [ ] SHARED A STORY
- [ ] WROTE A PERSONAL NOTE OR TEXT

REFLECT

HOW I'D RATE MY FEELING OF CONNECTION TODAY:

| 1 | 2 | 3 | 4 | 5 | 6 | 7 | 8 | 9 | 10 |

LONELY / DISCONNECTED   HIGHLY CONNECTED

THE MOST MEANINGFUL INTERACTION
I HAD TODAY AND HOW IT MADE ME FEEL:

_____
_____
_____
_____
_____
_____
_____
_____
_____

CHALLENGES TO DEVELOPING DEEPER BONDS
AND HOW I CAN OVERCOME THEM:

_____
_____
_____

WAYS I'D LIKE TO CONNECT MORE:

_____
_____
_____
_____

RECORD

DATE ___/___/___

MY GOALS FOR MEANINGFUL CONNECTIONS TODAY:

- [ ] _____
- [ ] _____
- [ ] _____

PEOPLE I'D LIKE TO CONNECT WITH:

_____
_____

WAYS TO STRENGTHEN MY RELATIONSHIPS:

_____
_____

WAYS I CONNECTED WITH OTHERS TODAY:

- [ ] CALLED A FRIEND
- [ ] ENCOURAGED SOMEONE
- [ ] ASKED FOR HELP OR ADVICE
- [ ] PLANNED ONE-ON-ONE TIME
- [ ] PRACTICED ACTIVE LISTENING
- [ ] EXPRESSED MY GRATITUDE TO SOMEONE ELSE
- [ ] SPENT QUALITY TIME WITH A FRIEND OR FAMILY MEMBER
- [ ] HELPED SOMEONE
- [ ] SHARED SOMETHING PERSONAL ABOUT MYSELF
- [ ] PRACTICED VULNERABILITY WITH A TRUSTED FRIEND
- [ ] SHARED A LAUGH
- [ ] TALKED TO SOMEONE NEW
- [ ] COMPLIMENTED SOMEONE
- [ ] COMPLETED A SHARED ACTIVITY
- [ ] NOTED SOMEONE ELSE'S MEANINGFUL DATE, EVENT, OR INTEREST I'D LIKE TO REMEMBER
- [ ] LET SOMEONE KNOW I WAS THINKING OF THEM
- [ ] PRACTICED BEING MORE PRESENT WITH OTHERS
- [ ] SHARED A STORY
- [ ] WROTE A PERSONAL NOTE OR TEXT

REFLECT

HOW I'D RATE MY FEELING OF CONNECTION TODAY:

| 1 | 2 | 3 | 4 | 5 | 6 | 7 | 8 | 9 | 10 |

LONELY / DISCONNECTED   HIGHLY CONNECTED

THE MOST MEANINGFUL INTERACTION
I HAD TODAY AND HOW IT MADE ME FEEL:

_____
_____
_____
_____
_____
_____
_____
_____

CHALLENGES TO DEVELOPING DEEPER BONDS
AND HOW I CAN OVERCOME THEM:

_____
_____
_____

WAYS I'D LIKE TO CONNECT MORE:

_____
_____
_____
_____

RECORD

DATE ___/___/___

MY GOALS FOR MEANINGFUL CONNECTIONS TODAY:

- ☐ _____
- ☐ _____
- ☐ _____

PEOPLE I'D LIKE TO CONNECT WITH:

_____
_____

WAYS TO STRENGTHEN MY RELATIONSHIPS:

_____
_____

WAYS I CONNECTED WITH OTHERS TODAY:

- ☐ CALLED A FRIEND
- ☐ ENCOURAGED SOMEONE
- ☐ ASKED FOR HELP OR ADVICE
- ☐ PLANNED ONE-ON-ONE TIME
- ☐ PRACTICED ACTIVE LISTENING
- ☐ EXPRESSED MY GRATITUDE TO SOMEONE ELSE
- ☐ SPENT QUALITY TIME WITH A FRIEND OR FAMILY MEMBER
- ☐ HELPED SOMEONE
- ☐ SHARED SOMETHING PERSONAL ABOUT MYSELF
- ☐ PRACTICED VULNERABILITY WITH A TRUSTED FRIEND
- ☐ SHARED A LAUGH
- ☐ TALKED TO SOMEONE NEW
- ☐ COMPLIMENTED SOMEONE
- ☐ COMPLETED A SHARED ACTIVITY
- ☐ NOTED SOMEONE ELSE'S MEANINGFUL DATE, EVENT, OR INTEREST I'D LIKE TO REMEMBER
- ☐ LET SOMEONE KNOW I WAS THINKING OF THEM
- ☐ PRACTICED BEING MORE PRESENT WITH OTHERS
- ☐ SHARED A STORY
- ☐ WROTE A PERSONAL NOTE OR TEXT

REFLECT

HOW I'D RATE MY FEELING OF CONNECTION TODAY:

| 1 | 2 | 3 | 4 | 5 | 6 | 7 | 8 | 9 | 10 |

LONELY / DISCONNECTED   HIGHLY CONNECTED

THE MOST MEANINGFUL INTERACTION
I HAD TODAY AND HOW IT MADE ME FEEL:

_____
_____
_____
_____
_____
_____
_____
_____

CHALLENGES TO DEVELOPING DEEPER BONDS
AND HOW I CAN OVERCOME THEM:

_____
_____
_____

WAYS I'D LIKE TO CONNECT MORE:

_____
_____
_____
_____

RECORD

DATE ___/___/___

MY GOALS FOR MEANINGFUL CONNECTIONS TODAY:

- [ ] _____
- [ ] _____
- [ ] _____

PEOPLE I'D LIKE TO CONNECT WITH:

_____
_____

WAYS TO STRENGTHEN MY RELATIONSHIPS:

_____
_____

WAYS I CONNECTED WITH OTHERS TODAY:

- [ ] CALLED A FRIEND
- [ ] ENCOURAGED SOMEONE
- [ ] ASKED FOR HELP OR ADVICE
- [ ] PLANNED ONE-ON-ONE TIME
- [ ] PRACTICED ACTIVE LISTENING
- [ ] EXPRESSED MY GRATITUDE TO SOMEONE ELSE
- [ ] SPENT QUALITY TIME WITH A FRIEND OR FAMILY MEMBER
- [ ] HELPED SOMEONE
- [ ] SHARED SOMETHING PERSONAL ABOUT MYSELF
- [ ] PRACTICED VULNERABILITY WITH A TRUSTED FRIEND

- [ ] SHARED A LAUGH
- [ ] TALKED TO SOMEONE NEW
- [ ] COMPLIMENTED SOMEONE
- [ ] COMPLETED A SHARED ACTIVITY
- [ ] NOTED SOMEONE ELSE'S MEANINGFUL DATE, EVENT, OR INTEREST I'D LIKE TO REMEMBER
- [ ] LET SOMEONE KNOW I WAS THINKING OF THEM
- [ ] PRACTICED BEING MORE PRESENT WITH OTHERS
- [ ] SHARED A STORY
- [ ] WROTE A PERSONAL NOTE OR TEXT

REFLECT

HOW I'D RATE MY FEELING OF CONNECTION TODAY:

| 1 | 2 | 3 | 4 | 5 | 6 | 7 | 8 | 9 | 10 |

LONELY / DISCONNECTED   HIGHLY CONNECTED

THE MOST MEANINGFUL INTERACTION
I HAD TODAY AND HOW IT MADE ME FEEL:

_____
_____
_____
_____
_____
_____
_____
_____
_____

CHALLENGES TO DEVELOPING DEEPER BONDS
AND HOW I CAN OVERCOME THEM:

_____
_____
_____

WAYS I'D LIKE TO CONNECT MORE:

_____
_____
_____
_____

RECORD

DATE ___/___/___

MY GOALS FOR MEANINGFUL CONNECTIONS TODAY:

- [ ] _____
- [ ] _____
- [ ] _____

PEOPLE I'D LIKE TO CONNECT WITH:

_____
_____

WAYS TO STRENGTHEN MY RELATIONSHIPS:

_____
_____

WAYS I CONNECTED WITH OTHERS TODAY:

- [ ] CALLED A FRIEND
- [ ] ENCOURAGED SOMEONE
- [ ] ASKED FOR HELP OR ADVICE
- [ ] PLANNED ONE-ON-ONE TIME
- [ ] PRACTICED ACTIVE LISTENING
- [ ] EXPRESSED MY GRATITUDE TO SOMEONE ELSE
- [ ] SPENT QUALITY TIME WITH A FRIEND OR FAMILY MEMBER
- [ ] HELPED SOMEONE
- [ ] SHARED SOMETHING PERSONAL ABOUT MYSELF
- [ ] PRACTICED VULNERABILITY WITH A TRUSTED FRIEND
- [ ] SHARED A LAUGH
- [ ] TALKED TO SOMEONE NEW
- [ ] COMPLIMENTED SOMEONE
- [ ] COMPLETED A SHARED ACTIVITY
- [ ] NOTED SOMEONE ELSE'S MEANINGFUL DATE, EVENT, OR INTEREST I'D LIKE TO REMEMBER
- [ ] LET SOMEONE KNOW I WAS THINKING OF THEM
- [ ] PRACTICED BEING MORE PRESENT WITH OTHERS
- [ ] SHARED A STORY
- [ ] WROTE A PERSONAL NOTE OR TEXT

REFLECT

HOW I'D RATE MY FEELING OF CONNECTION TODAY:

| 1 | 2 | 3 | 4 | 5 | 6 | 7 | 8 | 9 | 10 |

LONELY / DISCONNECTED   HIGHLY CONNECTED

THE MOST MEANINGFUL INTERACTION
I HAD TODAY AND HOW IT MADE ME FEEL:

_____
_____
_____
_____
_____
_____
_____
_____
_____

CHALLENGES TO DEVELOPING DEEPER BONDS
AND HOW I CAN OVERCOME THEM:

_____
_____
_____

WAYS I'D LIKE TO CONNECT MORE:

_____
_____
_____
_____

RECORD

DATE ___/___/___

MY GOALS FOR MEANINGFUL CONNECTIONS TODAY:

☐ _____
☐ _____
☐ _____

PEOPLE I'D LIKE TO CONNECT WITH:

_____
_____

WAYS TO STRENGTHEN MY RELATIONSHIPS:

_____
_____

WAYS I CONNECTED WITH OTHERS TODAY:

- ☐ CALLED A FRIEND
- ☐ ENCOURAGED SOMEONE
- ☐ ASKED FOR HELP OR ADVICE
- ☐ PLANNED ONE-ON-ONE TIME
- ☐ PRACTICED ACTIVE LISTENING
- ☐ EXPRESSED MY GRATITUDE TO SOMEONE ELSE
- ☐ SPENT QUALITY TIME WITH A FRIEND OR FAMILY MEMBER
- ☐ HELPED SOMEONE
- ☐ SHARED SOMETHING PERSONAL ABOUT MYSELF
- ☐ PRACTICED VULNERABILITY WITH A TRUSTED FRIEND
- ☐ SHARED A LAUGH
- ☐ TALKED TO SOMEONE NEW
- ☐ COMPLIMENTED SOMEONE
- ☐ COMPLETED A SHARED ACTIVITY
- ☐ NOTED SOMEONE ELSE'S MEANINGFUL DATE, EVENT, OR INTEREST I'D LIKE TO REMEMBER
- ☐ LET SOMEONE KNOW I WAS THINKING OF THEM
- ☐ PRACTICED BEING MORE PRESENT WITH OTHERS
- ☐ SHARED A STORY
- ☐ WROTE A PERSONAL NOTE OR TEXT

REFLECT

HOW I'D RATE MY FEELING OF CONNECTION TODAY:

| 1 | 2 | 3 | 4 | 5 | 6 | 7 | 8 | 9 | 10 |

LONELY / DISCONNECTED   HIGHLY CONNECTED

THE MOST MEANINGFUL INTERACTION
I HAD TODAY AND HOW IT MADE ME FEEL:

_____
_____
_____
_____
_____
_____
_____
_____

CHALLENGES TO DEVELOPING DEEPER BONDS
AND HOW I CAN OVERCOME THEM:

_____
_____
_____

WAYS I'D LIKE TO CONNECT MORE:

_____
_____
_____
_____

RECORD

DATE ___/___/___

MY GOALS FOR MEANINGFUL CONNECTIONS TODAY:

- [ ] _____
- [ ] _____
- [ ] _____

PEOPLE I'D LIKE TO CONNECT WITH:

_____
_____

WAYS TO STRENGTHEN MY RELATIONSHIPS:

_____
_____

WAYS I CONNECTED WITH OTHERS TODAY:

- [ ] CALLED A FRIEND
- [ ] ENCOURAGED SOMEONE
- [ ] ASKED FOR HELP OR ADVICE
- [ ] PLANNED ONE-ON-ONE TIME
- [ ] PRACTICED ACTIVE LISTENING
- [ ] EXPRESSED MY GRATITUDE TO SOMEONE ELSE
- [ ] SPENT QUALITY TIME WITH A FRIEND OR FAMILY MEMBER
- [ ] HELPED SOMEONE
- [ ] SHARED SOMETHING PERSONAL ABOUT MYSELF
- [ ] PRACTICED VULNERABILITY WITH A TRUSTED FRIEND
- [ ] SHARED A LAUGH
- [ ] TALKED TO SOMEONE NEW
- [ ] COMPLIMENTED SOMEONE
- [ ] COMPLETED A SHARED ACTIVITY
- [ ] NOTED SOMEONE ELSE'S MEANINGFUL DATE, EVENT, OR INTEREST I'D LIKE TO REMEMBER
- [ ] LET SOMEONE KNOW I WAS THINKING OF THEM
- [ ] PRACTICED BEING MORE PRESENT WITH OTHERS
- [ ] SHARED A STORY
- [ ] WROTE A PERSONAL NOTE OR TEXT

REFLECT

HOW I'D RATE MY FEELING OF CONNECTION TODAY:

| 1 | 2 | 3 | 4 | 5 | 6 | 7 | 8 | 9 | 10 |

LONELY / DISCONNECTED   HIGHLY CONNECTED

THE MOST MEANINGFUL INTERACTION
I HAD TODAY AND HOW IT MADE ME FEEL:

_____
_____
_____
_____
_____
_____
_____
_____
_____

CHALLENGES TO DEVELOPING DEEPER BONDS
AND HOW I CAN OVERCOME THEM:

_____
_____
_____

WAYS I'D LIKE TO CONNECT MORE:

_____
_____
_____
_____

RECORD

DATE ___/___/___

MY GOALS FOR MEANINGFUL CONNECTIONS TODAY:

- [ ] _____
- [ ] _____
- [ ] _____

PEOPLE I'D LIKE TO CONNECT WITH:

_____
_____

WAYS TO STRENGTHEN MY RELATIONSHIPS:

_____
_____

WAYS I CONNECTED WITH OTHERS TODAY:

- [ ] CALLED A FRIEND
- [ ] ENCOURAGED SOMEONE
- [ ] ASKED FOR HELP OR ADVICE
- [ ] PLANNED ONE-ON-ONE TIME
- [ ] PRACTICED ACTIVE LISTENING
- [ ] EXPRESSED MY GRATITUDE TO SOMEONE ELSE
- [ ] SPENT QUALITY TIME WITH A FRIEND OR FAMILY MEMBER
- [ ] HELPED SOMEONE
- [ ] SHARED SOMETHING PERSONAL ABOUT MYSELF
- [ ] PRACTICED VULNERABILITY WITH A TRUSTED FRIEND
- [ ] SHARED A LAUGH
- [ ] TALKED TO SOMEONE NEW
- [ ] COMPLIMENTED SOMEONE
- [ ] COMPLETED A SHARED ACTIVITY
- [ ] NOTED SOMEONE ELSE'S MEANINGFUL DATE, EVENT, OR INTEREST I'D LIKE TO REMEMBER
- [ ] LET SOMEONE KNOW I WAS THINKING OF THEM
- [ ] PRACTICED BEING MORE PRESENT WITH OTHERS
- [ ] SHARED A STORY
- [ ] WROTE A PERSONAL NOTE OR TEXT

REFLECT

HOW I'D RATE MY FEELING OF CONNECTION TODAY:

| 1 | 2 | 3 | 4 | 5 | 6 | 7 | 8 | 9 | 10 |

LONELY / DISCONNECTED   HIGHLY CONNECTED

THE MOST MEANINGFUL INTERACTION
I HAD TODAY AND HOW IT MADE ME FEEL:

_____
_____
_____
_____
_____
_____
_____
_____
_____

CHALLENGES TO DEVELOPING DEEPER BONDS
AND HOW I CAN OVERCOME THEM:

_____
_____
_____

WAYS I'D LIKE TO CONNECT MORE:

_____
_____
_____
_____

RECORD

DATE ___ / ___ / ___

MY GOALS FOR MEANINGFUL CONNECTIONS TODAY:

☐ _____
☐ _____
☐ _____

PEOPLE I'D LIKE TO CONNECT WITH:

_____
_____

WAYS TO STRENGTHEN MY RELATIONSHIPS:

_____
_____

WAYS I CONNECTED WITH OTHERS TODAY:

- ☐ CALLED A FRIEND
- ☐ ENCOURAGED SOMEONE
- ☐ ASKED FOR HELP OR ADVICE
- ☐ PLANNED ONE-ON-ONE TIME
- ☐ PRACTICED ACTIVE LISTENING
- ☐ EXPRESSED MY GRATITUDE TO SOMEONE ELSE
- ☐ SPENT QUALITY TIME WITH A FRIEND OR FAMILY MEMBER
- ☐ HELPED SOMEONE
- ☐ SHARED SOMETHING PERSONAL ABOUT MYSELF
- ☐ PRACTICED VULNERABILITY WITH A TRUSTED FRIEND
- ☐ SHARED A LAUGH
- ☐ TALKED TO SOMEONE NEW
- ☐ COMPLIMENTED SOMEONE
- ☐ COMPLETED A SHARED ACTIVITY
- ☐ NOTED SOMEONE ELSE'S MEANINGFUL DATE, EVENT, OR INTEREST I'D LIKE TO REMEMBER
- ☐ LET SOMEONE KNOW I WAS THINKING OF THEM
- ☐ PRACTICED BEING MORE PRESENT WITH OTHERS
- ☐ SHARED A STORY
- ☐ WROTE A PERSONAL NOTE OR TEXT

REFLECT

HOW I'D RATE MY FEELING OF CONNECTION TODAY:

| 1 | 2 | 3 | 4 | 5 | 6 | 7 | 8 | 9 | 10 |

LONELY / DISCONNECTED   HIGHLY CONNECTED

THE MOST MEANINGFUL INTERACTION
I HAD TODAY AND HOW IT MADE ME FEEL:

_____
_____
_____
_____
_____
_____
_____
_____

CHALLENGES TO DEVELOPING DEEPER BONDS
AND HOW I CAN OVERCOME THEM:

_____
_____
_____

WAYS I'D LIKE TO CONNECT MORE:

_____
_____
_____
_____

RECORD

DATE ___/___/___

MY GOALS FOR MEANINGFUL CONNECTIONS TODAY:
- ☐ _____
- ☐ _____
- ☐ _____

PEOPLE I'D LIKE TO CONNECT WITH:
_____
_____

WAYS TO STRENGTHEN MY RELATIONSHIPS:
_____
_____

WAYS I CONNECTED WITH OTHERS TODAY:

- ☐ CALLED A FRIEND
- ☐ ENCOURAGED SOMEONE
- ☐ ASKED FOR HELP OR ADVICE
- ☐ PLANNED ONE-ON-ONE TIME
- ☐ PRACTICED ACTIVE LISTENING
- ☐ EXPRESSED MY GRATITUDE TO SOMEONE ELSE
- ☐ SPENT QUALITY TIME WITH A FRIEND OR FAMILY MEMBER
- ☐ HELPED SOMEONE
- ☐ SHARED SOMETHING PERSONAL ABOUT MYSELF
- ☐ PRACTICED VULNERABILITY WITH A TRUSTED FRIEND
- ☐ SHARED A LAUGH
- ☐ TALKED TO SOMEONE NEW
- ☐ COMPLIMENTED SOMEONE
- ☐ COMPLETED A SHARED ACTIVITY
- ☐ NOTED SOMEONE ELSE'S MEANINGFUL DATE, EVENT, OR INTEREST I'D LIKE TO REMEMBER
- ☐ LET SOMEONE KNOW I WAS THINKING OF THEM
- ☐ PRACTICED BEING MORE PRESENT WITH OTHERS
- ☐ SHARED A STORY
- ☐ WROTE A PERSONAL NOTE OR TEXT

REFLECT

HOW I'D RATE MY FEELING OF CONNECTION TODAY:

| 1 | 2 | 3 | 4 | 5 | 6 | 7 | 8 | 9 | 10 |

LONELY / DISCONNECTED   HIGHLY CONNECTED

THE MOST MEANINGFUL INTERACTION
I HAD TODAY AND HOW IT MADE ME FEEL:
_____
_____
_____
_____
_____
_____
_____
_____
_____

CHALLENGES TO DEVELOPING DEEPER BONDS
AND HOW I CAN OVERCOME THEM:
_____
_____
_____

WAYS I'D LIKE TO CONNECT MORE:
_____
_____
_____
_____

RECORD

DATE ___/___/___

MY GOALS FOR MEANINGFUL CONNECTIONS TODAY:
- [ ] _____
- [ ] _____
- [ ] _____

PEOPLE I'D LIKE TO CONNECT WITH:
_____
_____

WAYS TO STRENGTHEN MY RELATIONSHIPS:
_____
_____

WAYS I CONNECTED WITH OTHERS TODAY:

- [ ] CALLED A FRIEND
- [ ] ENCOURAGED SOMEONE
- [ ] ASKED FOR HELP OR ADVICE
- [ ] PLANNED ONE-ON-ONE TIME
- [ ] PRACTICED ACTIVE LISTENING
- [ ] EXPRESSED MY GRATITUDE TO SOMEONE ELSE
- [ ] SPENT QUALITY TIME WITH A FRIEND OR FAMILY MEMBER
- [ ] HELPED SOMEONE
- [ ] SHARED SOMETHING PERSONAL ABOUT MYSELF
- [ ] PRACTICED VULNERABILITY WITH A TRUSTED FRIEND
- [ ] SHARED A LAUGH
- [ ] TALKED TO SOMEONE NEW
- [ ] COMPLIMENTED SOMEONE
- [ ] COMPLETED A SHARED ACTIVITY
- [ ] NOTED SOMEONE ELSE'S MEANINGFUL DATE, EVENT, OR INTEREST I'D LIKE TO REMEMBER
- [ ] LET SOMEONE KNOW I WAS THINKING OF THEM
- [ ] PRACTICED BEING MORE PRESENT WITH OTHERS
- [ ] SHARED A STORY
- [ ] WROTE A PERSONAL NOTE OR TEXT

REFLECT

HOW I'D RATE MY FEELING OF CONNECTION TODAY:

| 1 | 2 | 3 | 4 | 5 | 6 | 7 | 8 | 9 | 10 |

LONELY / DISCONNECTED   HIGHLY CONNECTED

THE MOST MEANINGFUL INTERACTION
I HAD TODAY AND HOW IT MADE ME FEEL:

_____
_____
_____
_____
_____
_____
_____
_____
_____

CHALLENGES TO DEVELOPING DEEPER BONDS
AND HOW I CAN OVERCOME THEM:

_____
_____
_____

WAYS I'D LIKE TO CONNECT MORE:

_____
_____
_____
_____

RECORD

DATE ___/___/___

MY GOALS FOR MEANINGFUL CONNECTIONS TODAY:

- [ ] _____
- [ ] _____
- [ ] _____

PEOPLE I'D LIKE TO CONNECT WITH:
_____
_____

WAYS TO STRENGTHEN MY RELATIONSHIPS:
_____
_____

WAYS I CONNECTED WITH OTHERS TODAY:

- [ ] CALLED A FRIEND
- [ ] ENCOURAGED SOMEONE
- [ ] ASKED FOR HELP OR ADVICE
- [ ] PLANNED ONE-ON-ONE TIME
- [ ] PRACTICED ACTIVE LISTENING
- [ ] EXPRESSED MY GRATITUDE TO SOMEONE ELSE
- [ ] SPENT QUALITY TIME WITH A FRIEND OR FAMILY MEMBER
- [ ] HELPED SOMEONE
- [ ] SHARED SOMETHING PERSONAL ABOUT MYSELF
- [ ] PRACTICED VULNERABILITY WITH A TRUSTED FRIEND
- [ ] SHARED A LAUGH
- [ ] TALKED TO SOMEONE NEW
- [ ] COMPLIMENTED SOMEONE
- [ ] COMPLETED A SHARED ACTIVITY
- [ ] NOTED SOMEONE ELSE'S MEANINGFUL DATE, EVENT, OR INTEREST I'D LIKE TO REMEMBER
- [ ] LET SOMEONE KNOW I WAS THINKING OF THEM
- [ ] PRACTICED BEING MORE PRESENT WITH OTHERS
- [ ] SHARED A STORY
- [ ] WROTE A PERSONAL NOTE OR TEXT

REFLECT

HOW I'D RATE MY FEELING OF CONNECTION TODAY:

| 1 | 2 | 3 | 4 | 5 | 6 | 7 | 8 | 9 | 10 |

LONELY / DISCONNECTED   HIGHLY CONNECTED

THE MOST MEANINGFUL INTERACTION
I HAD TODAY AND HOW IT MADE ME FEEL:

_____
_____
_____
_____
_____
_____
_____
_____
_____

CHALLENGES TO DEVELOPING DEEPER BONDS
AND HOW I CAN OVERCOME THEM:

_____
_____
_____

WAYS I'D LIKE TO CONNECT MORE:

_____
_____
_____
_____

RECORD

DATE ___/___/___

MY GOALS FOR MEANINGFUL CONNECTIONS TODAY:

- [ ] _____
- [ ] _____
- [ ] _____

PEOPLE I'D LIKE TO CONNECT WITH:

_____
_____

WAYS TO STRENGTHEN MY RELATIONSHIPS:

_____
_____

WAYS I CONNECTED WITH OTHERS TODAY:

- [ ] CALLED A FRIEND
- [ ] ENCOURAGED SOMEONE
- [ ] ASKED FOR HELP OR ADVICE
- [ ] PLANNED ONE-ON-ONE TIME
- [ ] PRACTICED ACTIVE LISTENING
- [ ] EXPRESSED MY GRATITUDE TO SOMEONE ELSE
- [ ] SPENT QUALITY TIME WITH A FRIEND OR FAMILY MEMBER
- [ ] HELPED SOMEONE
- [ ] SHARED SOMETHING PERSONAL ABOUT MYSELF
- [ ] PRACTICED VULNERABILITY WITH A TRUSTED FRIEND
- [ ] SHARED A LAUGH
- [ ] TALKED TO SOMEONE NEW
- [ ] COMPLIMENTED SOMEONE
- [ ] COMPLETED A SHARED ACTIVITY
- [ ] NOTED SOMEONE ELSE'S MEANINGFUL DATE, EVENT, OR INTEREST I'D LIKE TO REMEMBER
- [ ] LET SOMEONE KNOW I WAS THINKING OF THEM
- [ ] PRACTICED BEING MORE PRESENT WITH OTHERS
- [ ] SHARED A STORY
- [ ] WROTE A PERSONAL NOTE OR TEXT

REFLECT

HOW I'D RATE MY FEELING OF CONNECTION TODAY:

| 1 | 2 | 3 | 4 | 5 | 6 | 7 | 8 | 9 | 10 |

LONELY / DISCONNECTED   HIGHLY CONNECTED

THE MOST MEANINGFUL INTERACTION
I HAD TODAY AND HOW IT MADE ME FEEL:
_____
_____
_____
_____
_____
_____
_____
_____
_____

CHALLENGES TO DEVELOPING DEEPER BONDS
AND HOW I CAN OVERCOME THEM:
_____
_____
_____

WAYS I'D LIKE TO CONNECT MORE:
_____
_____
_____

RECORD

DATE ___/___/___

MY GOALS FOR MEANINGFUL CONNECTIONS TODAY:

- [ ] _____
- [ ] _____
- [ ] _____

PEOPLE I'D LIKE TO CONNECT WITH:

_____
_____

WAYS TO STRENGTHEN MY RELATIONSHIPS:

_____
_____

WAYS I CONNECTED WITH OTHERS TODAY:

- [ ] CALLED A FRIEND
- [ ] ENCOURAGED SOMEONE
- [ ] ASKED FOR HELP OR ADVICE
- [ ] PLANNED ONE-ON-ONE TIME
- [ ] PRACTICED ACTIVE LISTENING
- [ ] EXPRESSED MY GRATITUDE TO SOMEONE ELSE
- [ ] SPENT QUALITY TIME WITH A FRIEND OR FAMILY MEMBER
- [ ] HELPED SOMEONE
- [ ] SHARED SOMETHING PERSONAL ABOUT MYSELF
- [ ] PRACTICED VULNERABILITY WITH A TRUSTED FRIEND
- [ ] SHARED A LAUGH
- [ ] TALKED TO SOMEONE NEW
- [ ] COMPLIMENTED SOMEONE
- [ ] COMPLETED A SHARED ACTIVITY
- [ ] NOTED SOMEONE ELSE'S MEANINGFUL DATE, EVENT, OR INTEREST I'D LIKE TO REMEMBER
- [ ] LET SOMEONE KNOW I WAS THINKING OF THEM
- [ ] PRACTICED BEING MORE PRESENT WITH OTHERS
- [ ] SHARED A STORY
- [ ] WROTE A PERSONAL NOTE OR TEXT

REFLECT

HOW I'D RATE MY FEELING OF CONNECTION TODAY:

| 1 | 2 | 3 | 4 | 5 | 6 | 7 | 8 | 9 | 10 |

LONELY / DISCONNECTED   HIGHLY CONNECTED

THE MOST MEANINGFUL INTERACTION
I HAD TODAY AND HOW IT MADE ME FEEL:

_____
_____
_____
_____
_____
_____
_____
_____
_____

CHALLENGES TO DEVELOPING DEEPER BONDS
AND HOW I CAN OVERCOME THEM:

_____
_____
_____

WAYS I'D LIKE TO CONNECT MORE:

_____
_____
_____
_____

RECORD

DATE ___/___/___

MY GOALS FOR MEANINGFUL CONNECTIONS TODAY:

- ☐ _____
- ☐ _____
- ☐ _____

PEOPLE I'D LIKE TO CONNECT WITH:

_____
_____

WAYS TO STRENGTHEN MY RELATIONSHIPS:

_____
_____

WAYS I CONNECTED WITH OTHERS TODAY:

- ☐ CALLED A FRIEND
- ☐ ENCOURAGED SOMEONE
- ☐ ASKED FOR HELP OR ADVICE
- ☐ PLANNED ONE-ON-ONE TIME
- ☐ PRACTICED ACTIVE LISTENING
- ☐ EXPRESSED MY GRATITUDE TO SOMEONE ELSE
- ☐ SPENT QUALITY TIME WITH A FRIEND OR FAMILY MEMBER
- ☐ HELPED SOMEONE
- ☐ SHARED SOMETHING PERSONAL ABOUT MYSELF
- ☐ PRACTICED VULNERABILITY WITH A TRUSTED FRIEND
- ☐ SHARED A LAUGH
- ☐ TALKED TO SOMEONE NEW
- ☐ COMPLIMENTED SOMEONE
- ☐ COMPLETED A SHARED ACTIVITY
- ☐ NOTED SOMEONE ELSE'S MEANINGFUL DATE, EVENT, OR INTEREST I'D LIKE TO REMEMBER
- ☐ LET SOMEONE KNOW I WAS THINKING OF THEM
- ☐ PRACTICED BEING MORE PRESENT WITH OTHERS
- ☐ SHARED A STORY
- ☐ WROTE A PERSONAL NOTE OR TEXT

REFLECT

HOW I'D RATE MY FEELING OF CONNECTION TODAY:

| 1 | 2 | 3 | 4 | 5 | 6 | 7 | 8 | 9 | 10 |

LONELY / DISCONNECTED						HIGHLY CONNECTED

THE MOST MEANINGFUL INTERACTION
I HAD TODAY AND HOW IT MADE ME FEEL:
___
___
___
___
___
___
___
___
___
___

CHALLENGES TO DEVELOPING DEEPER BONDS
AND HOW I CAN OVERCOME THEM:
___
___
___

WAYS I'D LIKE TO CONNECT MORE:
___
___
___
___

RECORD

DATE ___/___/___

MY GOALS FOR MEANINGFUL CONNECTIONS TODAY:

- [ ] _____
- [ ] _____
- [ ] _____

PEOPLE I'D LIKE TO CONNECT WITH:
_____
_____

WAYS TO STRENGTHEN MY RELATIONSHIPS:
_____
_____

WAYS I CONNECTED WITH OTHERS TODAY:

- [ ] CALLED A FRIEND
- [ ] ENCOURAGED SOMEONE
- [ ] ASKED FOR HELP OR ADVICE
- [ ] PLANNED ONE-ON-ONE TIME
- [ ] PRACTICED ACTIVE LISTENING
- [ ] EXPRESSED MY GRATITUDE TO SOMEONE ELSE
- [ ] SPENT QUALITY TIME WITH A FRIEND OR FAMILY MEMBER
- [ ] HELPED SOMEONE
- [ ] SHARED SOMETHING PERSONAL ABOUT MYSELF
- [ ] PRACTICED VULNERABILITY WITH A TRUSTED FRIEND
- [ ] SHARED A LAUGH
- [ ] TALKED TO SOMEONE NEW
- [ ] COMPLIMENTED SOMEONE
- [ ] COMPLETED A SHARED ACTIVITY
- [ ] NOTED SOMEONE ELSE'S MEANINGFUL DATE, EVENT, OR INTEREST I'D LIKE TO REMEMBER
- [ ] LET SOMEONE KNOW I WAS THINKING OF THEM
- [ ] PRACTICED BEING MORE PRESENT WITH OTHERS
- [ ] SHARED A STORY
- [ ] WROTE A PERSONAL NOTE OR TEXT

REFLECT

HOW I'D RATE MY FEELING OF CONNECTION TODAY:

| 1 | 2 | 3 | 4 | 5 | 6 | 7 | 8 | 9 | 10 |

LONELY / DISCONNECTED   HIGHLY CONNECTED

THE MOST MEANINGFUL INTERACTION
I HAD TODAY AND HOW IT MADE ME FEEL:

___

CHALLENGES TO DEVELOPING DEEPER BONDS
AND HOW I CAN OVERCOME THEM:

___

WAYS I'D LIKE TO CONNECT MORE:

RECORD

DATE ___/___/___

MY GOALS FOR MEANINGFUL CONNECTIONS TODAY:

- ☐ _____
- ☐ _____
- ☐ _____

PEOPLE I'D LIKE TO CONNECT WITH:
_____
_____

WAYS TO STRENGTHEN MY RELATIONSHIPS:
_____
_____

WAYS I CONNECTED WITH OTHERS TODAY:

- ☐ CALLED A FRIEND
- ☐ ENCOURAGED SOMEONE
- ☐ ASKED FOR HELP OR ADVICE
- ☐ PLANNED ONE-ON-ONE TIME
- ☐ PRACTICED ACTIVE LISTENING
- ☐ EXPRESSED MY GRATITUDE TO SOMEONE ELSE
- ☐ SPENT QUALITY TIME WITH A FRIEND OR FAMILY MEMBER
- ☐ HELPED SOMEONE
- ☐ SHARED SOMETHING PERSONAL ABOUT MYSELF
- ☐ PRACTICED VULNERABILITY WITH A TRUSTED FRIEND
- ☐ SHARED A LAUGH
- ☐ TALKED TO SOMEONE NEW
- ☐ COMPLIMENTED SOMEONE
- ☐ COMPLETED A SHARED ACTIVITY
- ☐ NOTED SOMEONE ELSE'S MEANINGFUL DATE, EVENT, OR INTEREST I'D LIKE TO REMEMBER
- ☐ LET SOMEONE KNOW I WAS THINKING OF THEM
- ☐ PRACTICED BEING MORE PRESENT WITH OTHERS
- ☐ SHARED A STORY
- ☐ WROTE A PERSONAL NOTE OR TEXT

REFLECT

HOW I'D RATE MY FEELING OF CONNECTION TODAY:

| 1 | 2 | 3 | 4 | 5 | 6 | 7 | 8 | 9 | 10 |

LONELY / DISCONNECTED   HIGHLY CONNECTED

THE MOST MEANINGFUL INTERACTION
I HAD TODAY AND HOW IT MADE ME FEEL:

_____
_____
_____
_____
_____
_____
_____
_____

CHALLENGES TO DEVELOPING DEEPER BONDS
AND HOW I CAN OVERCOME THEM:

_____
_____
_____
_____

WAYS I'D LIKE TO CONNECT MORE:

_____
_____
_____
_____

RECORD

DATE ___/___/___

MY GOALS FOR MEANINGFUL CONNECTIONS TODAY:

- [ ] _____
- [ ] _____
- [ ] _____

PEOPLE I'D LIKE TO CONNECT WITH:

_____
_____

WAYS TO STRENGTHEN MY RELATIONSHIPS:

_____
_____

WAYS I CONNECTED WITH OTHERS TODAY:

- [ ] CALLED A FRIEND
- [ ] ENCOURAGED SOMEONE
- [ ] ASKED FOR HELP OR ADVICE
- [ ] PLANNED ONE-ON-ONE TIME
- [ ] PRACTICED ACTIVE LISTENING
- [ ] EXPRESSED MY GRATITUDE TO SOMEONE ELSE
- [ ] SPENT QUALITY TIME WITH A FRIEND OR FAMILY MEMBER
- [ ] HELPED SOMEONE
- [ ] SHARED SOMETHING PERSONAL ABOUT MYSELF
- [ ] PRACTICED VULNERABILITY WITH A TRUSTED FRIEND
- [ ] SHARED A LAUGH
- [ ] TALKED TO SOMEONE NEW
- [ ] COMPLIMENTED SOMEONE
- [ ] COMPLETED A SHARED ACTIVITY
- [ ] NOTED SOMEONE ELSE'S MEANINGFUL DATE, EVENT, OR INTEREST I'D LIKE TO REMEMBER
- [ ] LET SOMEONE KNOW I WAS THINKING OF THEM
- [ ] PRACTICED BEING MORE PRESENT WITH OTHERS
- [ ] SHARED A STORY
- [ ] WROTE A PERSONAL NOTE OR TEXT

REFLECT

HOW I'D RATE MY FEELING OF CONNECTION TODAY:

| 1 | 2 | 3 | 4 | 5 | 6 | 7 | 8 | 9 | 10 |

LONELY / DISCONNECTED   HIGHLY CONNECTED

THE MOST MEANINGFUL INTERACTION
I HAD TODAY AND HOW IT MADE ME FEEL:

_____
_____
_____
_____
_____
_____
_____
_____

CHALLENGES TO DEVELOPING DEEPER BONDS
AND HOW I CAN OVERCOME THEM:

_____
_____
_____
_____

WAYS I'D LIKE TO CONNECT MORE:

_____
_____
_____
_____
_____

RECORD

DATE ___/___/___

MY GOALS FOR MEANINGFUL CONNECTIONS TODAY:
- ☐ _____
- ☐ _____
- ☐ _____

PEOPLE I'D LIKE TO CONNECT WITH:
_____
_____

WAYS TO STRENGTHEN MY RELATIONSHIPS:
_____
_____

WAYS I CONNECTED WITH OTHERS TODAY:

- ☐ CALLED A FRIEND
- ☐ ENCOURAGED SOMEONE
- ☐ ASKED FOR HELP OR ADVICE
- ☐ PLANNED ONE-ON-ONE TIME
- ☐ PRACTICED ACTIVE LISTENING
- ☐ EXPRESSED MY GRATITUDE TO SOMEONE ELSE
- ☐ SPENT QUALITY TIME WITH A FRIEND OR FAMILY MEMBER
- ☐ HELPED SOMEONE
- ☐ SHARED SOMETHING PERSONAL ABOUT MYSELF
- ☐ PRACTICED VULNERABILITY WITH A TRUSTED FRIEND
- ☐ SHARED A LAUGH
- ☐ TALKED TO SOMEONE NEW
- ☐ COMPLIMENTED SOMEONE
- ☐ COMPLETED A SHARED ACTIVITY
- ☐ NOTED SOMEONE ELSE'S MEANINGFUL DATE, EVENT, OR INTEREST I'D LIKE TO REMEMBER
- ☐ LET SOMEONE KNOW I WAS THINKING OF THEM
- ☐ PRACTICED BEING MORE PRESENT WITH OTHERS
- ☐ SHARED A STORY
- ☐ WROTE A PERSONAL NOTE OR TEXT

REFLECT

HOW I'D RATE MY FEELING OF CONNECTION TODAY:

| 1 | 2 | 3 | 4 | 5 | 6 | 7 | 8 | 9 | 10 |

LONELY / DISCONNECTED   HIGHLY CONNECTED

THE MOST MEANINGFUL INTERACTION
I HAD TODAY AND HOW IT MADE ME FEEL:

_____
_____
_____
_____
_____
_____
_____
_____

CHALLENGES TO DEVELOPING DEEPER BONDS
AND HOW I CAN OVERCOME THEM:

_____
_____
_____
_____

WAYS I'D LIKE TO CONNECT MORE:

_____
_____
_____
_____

RECORD

DATE ___ / ___ / ___

MY GOALS FOR MEANINGFUL CONNECTIONS TODAY:

☐ _____
☐ _____
☐ _____

PEOPLE I'D LIKE TO CONNECT WITH:

_____
_____

WAYS TO STRENGTHEN MY RELATIONSHIPS:

_____
_____

WAYS I CONNECTED WITH OTHERS TODAY:

- ☐ CALLED A FRIEND
- ☐ ENCOURAGED SOMEONE
- ☐ ASKED FOR HELP OR ADVICE
- ☐ PLANNED ONE-ON-ONE TIME
- ☐ PRACTICED ACTIVE LISTENING
- ☐ EXPRESSED MY GRATITUDE TO SOMEONE ELSE
- ☐ SPENT QUALITY TIME WITH A FRIEND OR FAMILY MEMBER
- ☐ HELPED SOMEONE
- ☐ SHARED SOMETHING PERSONAL ABOUT MYSELF
- ☐ PRACTICED VULNERABILITY WITH A TRUSTED FRIEND
- ☐ SHARED A LAUGH
- ☐ TALKED TO SOMEONE NEW
- ☐ COMPLIMENTED SOMEONE
- ☐ COMPLETED A SHARED ACTIVITY
- ☐ NOTED SOMEONE ELSE'S MEANINGFUL DATE, EVENT, OR INTEREST I'D LIKE TO REMEMBER
- ☐ LET SOMEONE KNOW I WAS THINKING OF THEM
- ☐ PRACTICED BEING MORE PRESENT WITH OTHERS
- ☐ SHARED A STORY
- ☐ WROTE A PERSONAL NOTE OR TEXT

REFLECT

HOW I'D RATE MY FEELING OF CONNECTION TODAY:

| 1 | 2 | 3 | 4 | 5 | 6 | 7 | 8 | 9 | 10 |

LONELY / DISCONNECTED   HIGHLY CONNECTED

THE MOST MEANINGFUL INTERACTION
I HAD TODAY AND HOW IT MADE ME FEEL:

_____
_____
_____
_____
_____
_____
_____
_____

CHALLENGES TO DEVELOPING DEEPER BONDS
AND HOW I CAN OVERCOME THEM:

_____
_____
_____
_____

WAYS I'D LIKE TO CONNECT MORE:

_____
_____
_____
_____

RECORD

DATE ____/____/____

MY GOALS FOR MEANINGFUL CONNECTIONS TODAY:

- ☐ _____
- ☐ _____
- ☐ _____

PEOPLE I'D LIKE TO CONNECT WITH:

_____
_____

WAYS TO STRENGTHEN MY RELATIONSHIPS:

_____
_____

WAYS I CONNECTED WITH OTHERS TODAY:

- ☐ CALLED A FRIEND
- ☐ ENCOURAGED SOMEONE
- ☐ ASKED FOR HELP OR ADVICE
- ☐ PLANNED ONE-ON-ONE TIME
- ☐ PRACTICED ACTIVE LISTENING
- ☐ EXPRESSED MY GRATITUDE TO SOMEONE ELSE
- ☐ SPENT QUALITY TIME WITH A FRIEND OR FAMILY MEMBER
- ☐ HELPED SOMEONE
- ☐ SHARED SOMETHING PERSONAL ABOUT MYSELF
- ☐ PRACTICED VULNERABILITY WITH A TRUSTED FRIEND
- ☐ SHARED A LAUGH
- ☐ TALKED TO SOMEONE NEW
- ☐ COMPLIMENTED SOMEONE
- ☐ COMPLETED A SHARED ACTIVITY
- ☐ NOTED SOMEONE ELSE'S MEANINGFUL DATE, EVENT, OR INTEREST I'D LIKE TO REMEMBER
- ☐ LET SOMEONE KNOW I WAS THINKING OF THEM
- ☐ PRACTICED BEING MORE PRESENT WITH OTHERS
- ☐ SHARED A STORY
- ☐ WROTE A PERSONAL NOTE OR TEXT

REFLECT

HOW I'D RATE MY FEELING OF CONNECTION TODAY:

| 1 | 2 | 3 | 4 | 5 | 6 | 7 | 8 | 9 | 10 |

LONELY / DISCONNECTED — HIGHLY CONNECTED

THE MOST MEANINGFUL INTERACTION
I HAD TODAY AND HOW IT MADE ME FEEL:
_____
_____
_____
_____
_____
_____
_____
_____

CHALLENGES TO DEVELOPING DEEPER BONDS
AND HOW I CAN OVERCOME THEM:
_____
_____
_____
_____

WAYS I'D LIKE TO CONNECT MORE:
_____
_____
_____
_____
_____

RECORD

DATE ___/___/___

MY GOALS FOR MEANINGFUL CONNECTIONS TODAY:
- ☐ _____
- ☐ _____
- ☐ _____

PEOPLE I'D LIKE TO CONNECT WITH:
_____
_____

WAYS TO STRENGTHEN MY RELATIONSHIPS:
_____
_____

WAYS I CONNECTED WITH OTHERS TODAY:

- ☐ CALLED A FRIEND
- ☐ ENCOURAGED SOMEONE
- ☐ ASKED FOR HELP OR ADVICE
- ☐ PLANNED ONE-ON-ONE TIME
- ☐ PRACTICED ACTIVE LISTENING
- ☐ EXPRESSED MY GRATITUDE TO SOMEONE ELSE
- ☐ SPENT QUALITY TIME WITH A FRIEND OR FAMILY MEMBER
- ☐ HELPED SOMEONE
- ☐ SHARED SOMETHING PERSONAL ABOUT MYSELF
- ☐ PRACTICED VULNERABILITY WITH A TRUSTED FRIEND
- ☐ SHARED A LAUGH
- ☐ TALKED TO SOMEONE NEW
- ☐ COMPLIMENTED SOMEONE
- ☐ COMPLETED A SHARED ACTIVITY
- ☐ NOTED SOMEONE ELSE'S MEANINGFUL DATE, EVENT, OR INTEREST I'D LIKE TO REMEMBER
- ☐ LET SOMEONE KNOW I WAS THINKING OF THEM
- ☐ PRACTICED BEING MORE PRESENT WITH OTHERS
- ☐ SHARED A STORY
- ☐ WROTE A PERSONAL NOTE OR TEXT

REFLECT

HOW I'D RATE MY FEELING OF CONNECTION TODAY:

| 1 | 2 | 3 | 4 | 5 | 6 | 7 | 8 | 9 | 10 |

LONELY / DISCONNECTED   HIGHLY CONNECTED

THE MOST MEANINGFUL INTERACTION
I HAD TODAY AND HOW IT MADE ME FEEL:

_____
_____
_____
_____
_____
_____
_____
_____
_____

CHALLENGES TO DEVELOPING DEEPER BONDS
AND HOW I CAN OVERCOME THEM:

_____
_____
_____
_____

WAYS I'D LIKE TO CONNECT MORE:

_____
_____
_____
_____

RECORD

DATE ___/___/___

MY GOALS FOR MEANINGFUL CONNECTIONS TODAY:
- ☐ _____
- ☐ _____
- ☐ _____

PEOPLE I'D LIKE TO CONNECT WITH:
_____
_____

WAYS TO STRENGTHEN MY RELATIONSHIPS:
_____
_____

WAYS I CONNECTED WITH OTHERS TODAY:

- ☐ CALLED A FRIEND
- ☐ ENCOURAGED SOMEONE
- ☐ ASKED FOR HELP OR ADVICE
- ☐ PLANNED ONE-ON-ONE TIME
- ☐ PRACTICED ACTIVE LISTENING
- ☐ EXPRESSED MY GRATITUDE TO SOMEONE ELSE
- ☐ SPENT QUALITY TIME WITH A FRIEND OR FAMILY MEMBER
- ☐ HELPED SOMEONE
- ☐ SHARED SOMETHING PERSONAL ABOUT MYSELF
- ☐ PRACTICED VULNERABILITY WITH A TRUSTED FRIEND
- ☐ SHARED A LAUGH
- ☐ TALKED TO SOMEONE NEW
- ☐ COMPLIMENTED SOMEONE
- ☐ COMPLETED A SHARED ACTIVITY
- ☐ NOTED SOMEONE ELSE'S MEANINGFUL DATE, EVENT, OR INTEREST I'D LIKE TO REMEMBER
- ☐ LET SOMEONE KNOW I WAS THINKING OF THEM
- ☐ PRACTICED BEING MORE PRESENT WITH OTHERS
- ☐ SHARED A STORY
- ☐ WROTE A PERSONAL NOTE OR TEXT

REFLECT

HOW I'D RATE MY FEELING OF CONNECTION TODAY:

| 1 | 2 | 3 | 4 | 5 | 6 | 7 | 8 | 9 | 10 |

LONELY / DISCONNECTED   HIGHLY CONNECTED

THE MOST MEANINGFUL INTERACTION
I HAD TODAY AND HOW IT MADE ME FEEL:

_____
_____
_____
_____
_____
_____
_____

CHALLENGES TO DEVELOPING DEEPER BONDS
AND HOW I CAN OVERCOME THEM:

_____
_____
_____
_____

WAYS I'D LIKE TO CONNECT MORE:

_____
_____
_____
_____
_____

RECORD

DATE ___/___/___

MY GOALS FOR MEANINGFUL CONNECTIONS TODAY:

- [ ] _____
- [ ] _____
- [ ] _____

PEOPLE I'D LIKE TO CONNECT WITH:

_____
_____

WAYS TO STRENGTHEN MY RELATIONSHIPS:

_____
_____

WAYS I CONNECTED WITH OTHERS TODAY:

- [ ] CALLED A FRIEND
- [ ] ENCOURAGED SOMEONE
- [ ] ASKED FOR HELP OR ADVICE
- [ ] PLANNED ONE-ON-ONE TIME
- [ ] PRACTICED ACTIVE LISTENING
- [ ] EXPRESSED MY GRATITUDE TO SOMEONE ELSE
- [ ] SPENT QUALITY TIME WITH A FRIEND OR FAMILY MEMBER
- [ ] HELPED SOMEONE
- [ ] SHARED SOMETHING PERSONAL ABOUT MYSELF
- [ ] PRACTICED VULNERABILITY WITH A TRUSTED FRIEND
- [ ] SHARED A LAUGH
- [ ] TALKED TO SOMEONE NEW
- [ ] COMPLIMENTED SOMEONE
- [ ] COMPLETED A SHARED ACTIVITY
- [ ] NOTED SOMEONE ELSE'S MEANINGFUL DATE, EVENT, OR INTEREST I'D LIKE TO REMEMBER
- [ ] LET SOMEONE KNOW I WAS THINKING OF THEM
- [ ] PRACTICED BEING MORE PRESENT WITH OTHERS
- [ ] SHARED A STORY
- [ ] WROTE A PERSONAL NOTE OR TEXT

REFLECT

HOW I'D RATE MY FEELING OF CONNECTION TODAY:

| 1 | 2 | 3 | 4 | 5 | 6 | 7 | 8 | 9 | 10 |

LONELY / DISCONNECTED   HIGHLY CONNECTED

THE MOST MEANINGFUL INTERACTION
I HAD TODAY AND HOW IT MADE ME FEEL:

_____
_____
_____
_____
_____
_____
_____
_____

CHALLENGES TO DEVELOPING DEEPER BONDS
AND HOW I CAN OVERCOME THEM:

_____
_____
_____
_____

WAYS I'D LIKE TO CONNECT MORE:

_____
_____
_____
_____

RECORD

DATE ___/___/___

MY GOALS FOR MEANINGFUL CONNECTIONS TODAY:
- ☐ _____
- ☐ _____
- ☐ _____

PEOPLE I'D LIKE TO CONNECT WITH:
_____
_____

WAYS TO STRENGTHEN MY RELATIONSHIPS:
_____
_____

WAYS I CONNECTED WITH OTHERS TODAY:

- ☐ CALLED A FRIEND
- ☐ ENCOURAGED SOMEONE
- ☐ ASKED FOR HELP OR ADVICE
- ☐ PLANNED ONE-ON-ONE TIME
- ☐ PRACTICED ACTIVE LISTENING
- ☐ EXPRESSED MY GRATITUDE TO SOMEONE ELSE
- ☐ SPENT QUALITY TIME WITH A FRIEND OR FAMILY MEMBER
- ☐ HELPED SOMEONE
- ☐ SHARED SOMETHING PERSONAL ABOUT MYSELF
- ☐ PRACTICED VULNERABILITY WITH A TRUSTED FRIEND

- ☐ SHARED A LAUGH
- ☐ TALKED TO SOMEONE NEW
- ☐ COMPLIMENTED SOMEONE
- ☐ COMPLETED A SHARED ACTIVITY
- ☐ NOTED SOMEONE ELSE'S MEANINGFUL DATE, EVENT, OR INTEREST I'D LIKE TO REMEMBER
- ☐ LET SOMEONE KNOW I WAS THINKING OF THEM
- ☐ PRACTICED BEING MORE PRESENT WITH OTHERS
- ☐ SHARED A STORY
- ☐ WROTE A PERSONAL NOTE OR TEXT

REFLECT

HOW I'D RATE MY FEELING OF CONNECTION TODAY:

1 2 3 4 5 6 7 8 9 10

LONELY / DISCONNECTED   HIGHLY CONNECTED

THE MOST MEANINGFUL INTERACTION
I HAD TODAY AND HOW IT MADE ME FEEL:

_____
_____
_____
_____
_____
_____
_____
_____

CHALLENGES TO DEVELOPING DEEPER BONDS
AND HOW I CAN OVERCOME THEM:

_____
_____
_____
_____
_____

WAYS I'D LIKE TO CONNECT MORE:

_____
_____
_____
_____
_____

RECORD

DATE ___ / ___ / ___

MY GOALS FOR MEANINGFUL CONNECTIONS TODAY:

- ☐ _____
- ☐ _____
- ☐ _____

PEOPLE I'D LIKE TO CONNECT WITH:

_____
_____

WAYS TO STRENGTHEN MY RELATIONSHIPS:

_____
_____

WAYS I CONNECTED WITH OTHERS TODAY:

- ☐ CALLED A FRIEND
- ☐ ENCOURAGED SOMEONE
- ☐ ASKED FOR HELP OR ADVICE
- ☐ PLANNED ONE-ON-ONE TIME
- ☐ PRACTICED ACTIVE LISTENING
- ☐ EXPRESSED MY GRATITUDE TO SOMEONE ELSE
- ☐ SPENT QUALITY TIME WITH A FRIEND OR FAMILY MEMBER
- ☐ HELPED SOMEONE.
- ☐ SHARED SOMETHING PERSONAL ABOUT MYSELF
- ☐ PRACTICED VULNERABILITY WITH A TRUSTED FRIEND
- ☐ SHARED A LAUGH
- ☐ TALKED TO SOMEONE NEW
- ☐ COMPLIMENTED SOMEONE
- ☐ COMPLETED A SHARED ACTIVITY
- ☐ NOTED SOMEONE ELSE'S MEANINGFUL DATE, EVENT, OR INTEREST I'D LIKE TO REMEMBER
- ☐ LET SOMEONE KNOW I WAS THINKING OF THEM
- ☐ PRACTICED BEING MORE PRESENT WITH OTHERS
- ☐ SHARED A STORY
- ☐ WROTE A PERSONAL NOTE OR TEXT

REFLECT

HOW I'D RATE MY FEELING OF CONNECTION TODAY:

| 1 | 2 | 3 | 4 | 5 | 6 | 7 | 8 | 9 | 10 |

LONELY / DISCONNECTED   HIGHLY CONNECTED

THE MOST MEANINGFUL INTERACTION
I HAD TODAY AND HOW IT MADE ME FEEL:

_____
_____
_____
_____
_____
_____
_____
_____

CHALLENGES TO DEVELOPING DEEPER BONDS
AND HOW I CAN OVERCOME THEM:

_____
_____
_____
_____

WAYS I'D LIKE TO CONNECT MORE:

_____
_____
_____
_____
_____

RECORD

DATE ___/___/___

MY GOALS FOR MEANINGFUL CONNECTIONS TODAY:
- ☐ _____
- ☐ _____
- ☐ _____

PEOPLE I'D LIKE TO CONNECT WITH:
_____
_____

WAYS TO STRENGTHEN MY RELATIONSHIPS:
_____
_____

WAYS I CONNECTED WITH OTHERS TODAY:

- ☐ CALLED A FRIEND
- ☐ ENCOURAGED SOMEONE
- ☐ ASKED FOR HELP OR ADVICE
- ☐ PLANNED ONE-ON-ONE TIME
- ☐ PRACTICED ACTIVE LISTENING
- ☐ EXPRESSED MY GRATITUDE TO SOMEONE ELSE
- ☐ SPENT QUALITY TIME WITH A FRIEND OR FAMILY MEMBER
- ☐ HELPED SOMEONE
- ☐ SHARED SOMETHING PERSONAL ABOUT MYSELF
- ☐ PRACTICED VULNERABILITY WITH A TRUSTED FRIEND
- ☐ SHARED A LAUGH
- ☐ TALKED TO SOMEONE NEW
- ☐ COMPLIMENTED SOMEONE
- ☐ COMPLETED A SHARED ACTIVITY
- ☐ NOTED SOMEONE ELSE'S MEANINGFUL DATE, EVENT, OR INTEREST I'D LIKE TO REMEMBER
- ☐ LET SOMEONE KNOW I WAS THINKING OF THEM
- ☐ PRACTICED BEING MORE PRESENT WITH OTHERS
- ☐ SHARED A STORY
- ☐ WROTE A PERSONAL NOTE OR TEXT

REFLECT

HOW I'D RATE MY FEELING OF CONNECTION TODAY:

| 1 | 2 | 3 | 4 | 5 | 6 | 7 | 8 | 9 | 10 |

LONELY / DISCONNECTED   HIGHLY CONNECTED

THE MOST MEANINGFUL INTERACTION
I HAD TODAY AND HOW IT MADE ME FEEL:

_____
_____
_____
_____
_____
_____
_____
_____
_____

CHALLENGES TO DEVELOPING DEEPER BONDS
AND HOW I CAN OVERCOME THEM:

_____
_____
_____
_____

WAYS I'D LIKE TO CONNECT MORE:

_____
_____
_____
_____
_____

RECORD

DATE ___/___/___

MY GOALS FOR MEANINGFUL CONNECTIONS TODAY:

- [ ] _____
- [ ] _____
- [ ] _____

PEOPLE I'D LIKE TO CONNECT WITH:

_____
_____

WAYS TO STRENGTHEN MY RELATIONSHIPS:

_____
_____

WAYS I CONNECTED WITH OTHERS TODAY:

- [ ] CALLED A FRIEND
- [ ] ENCOURAGED SOMEONE
- [ ] ASKED FOR HELP OR ADVICE
- [ ] PLANNED ONE-ON-ONE TIME
- [ ] PRACTICED ACTIVE LISTENING
- [ ] EXPRESSED MY GRATITUDE TO SOMEONE ELSE
- [ ] SPENT QUALITY TIME WITH A FRIEND OR FAMILY MEMBER
- [ ] HELPED SOMEONE
- [ ] SHARED SOMETHING PERSONAL ABOUT MYSELF
- [ ] PRACTICED VULNERABILITY WITH A TRUSTED FRIEND
- [ ] SHARED A LAUGH
- [ ] TALKED TO SOMEONE NEW
- [ ] COMPLIMENTED SOMEONE
- [ ] COMPLETED A SHARED ACTIVITY
- [ ] NOTED SOMEONE ELSE'S MEANINGFUL DATE, EVENT, OR INTEREST I'D LIKE TO REMEMBER
- [ ] LET SOMEONE KNOW I WAS THINKING OF THEM
- [ ] PRACTICED BEING MORE PRESENT WITH OTHERS
- [ ] SHARED A STORY
- [ ] WROTE A PERSONAL NOTE OR TEXT

REFLECT

HOW I'D RATE MY FEELING OF CONNECTION TODAY:

| 1 | 2 | 3 | 4 | 5 | 6 | 7 | 8 | 9 | 10 |

LONELY / DISCONNECTED   HIGHLY CONNECTED

THE MOST MEANINGFUL INTERACTION
I HAD TODAY AND HOW IT MADE ME FEEL:

_____
_____
_____
_____
_____
_____
_____
_____

CHALLENGES TO DEVELOPING DEEPER BONDS
AND HOW I CAN OVERCOME THEM:

_____
_____
_____
_____

WAYS I'D LIKE TO CONNECT MORE:

_____
_____
_____
_____
_____

RECORD

DATE ____/____/____

MY GOALS FOR MEANINGFUL CONNECTIONS TODAY:

- ☐ _____
- ☐ _____
- ☐ _____

PEOPLE I'D LIKE TO CONNECT WITH:

_____
_____

WAYS TO STRENGTHEN MY RELATIONSHIPS:

_____
_____

WAYS I CONNECTED WITH OTHERS TODAY:

- ☐ CALLED A FRIEND
- ☐ ENCOURAGED SOMEONE
- ☐ ASKED FOR HELP OR ADVICE
- ☐ PLANNED ONE-ON-ONE TIME
- ☐ PRACTICED ACTIVE LISTENING
- ☐ EXPRESSED MY GRATITUDE TO SOMEONE ELSE
- ☐ SPENT QUALITY TIME WITH A FRIEND OR FAMILY MEMBER
- ☐ HELPED SOMEONE
- ☐ SHARED SOMETHING PERSONAL ABOUT MYSELF
- ☐ PRACTICED VULNERABILITY WITH A TRUSTED FRIEND
- ☐ SHARED A LAUGH
- ☐ TALKED TO SOMEONE NEW
- ☐ COMPLIMENTED SOMEONE
- ☐ COMPLETED A SHARED ACTIVITY
- ☐ NOTED SOMEONE ELSE'S MEANINGFUL DATE, EVENT, OR INTEREST I'D LIKE TO REMEMBER
- ☐ LET SOMEONE KNOW I WAS THINKING OF THEM
- ☐ PRACTICED BEING MORE PRESENT WITH OTHERS
- ☐ SHARED A STORY
- ☐ WROTE A PERSONAL NOTE OR TEXT

REFLECT

HOW I'D RATE MY FEELING OF CONNECTION TODAY:

| 1 | 2 | 3 | 4 | 5 | 6 | 7 | 8 | 9 | 10 |

LONELY / DISCONNECTED   HIGHLY CONNECTED

THE MOST MEANINGFUL INTERACTION
I HAD TODAY AND HOW IT MADE ME FEEL:
___
___
___
___
___
___
___
___

CHALLENGES TO DEVELOPING DEEPER BONDS
AND HOW I CAN OVERCOME THEM:
___
___
___
___

WAYS I'D LIKE TO CONNECT MORE:
___
___
___
___
___

RECORD

DATE ___/___/___

MY GOALS FOR MEANINGFUL CONNECTIONS TODAY:

- [ ] _____
- [ ] _____
- [ ] _____

PEOPLE I'D LIKE TO CONNECT WITH:

_____
_____

WAYS TO STRENGTHEN MY RELATIONSHIPS:

_____
_____

WAYS I CONNECTED WITH OTHERS TODAY:

- [ ] CALLED A FRIEND
- [ ] ENCOURAGED SOMEONE
- [ ] ASKED FOR HELP OR ADVICE
- [ ] PLANNED ONE-ON-ONE TIME
- [ ] PRACTICED ACTIVE LISTENING
- [ ] EXPRESSED MY GRATITUDE TO SOMEONE ELSE
- [ ] SPENT QUALITY TIME WITH A FRIEND OR FAMILY MEMBER
- [ ] HELPED SOMEONE
- [ ] SHARED SOMETHING PERSONAL ABOUT MYSELF
- [ ] PRACTICED VULNERABILITY WITH A TRUSTED FRIEND
- [ ] SHARED A LAUGH
- [ ] TALKED TO SOMEONE NEW
- [ ] COMPLIMENTED SOMEONE
- [ ] COMPLETED A SHARED ACTIVITY
- [ ] NOTED SOMEONE ELSE'S MEANINGFUL DATE, EVENT, OR INTEREST I'D LIKE TO REMEMBER
- [ ] LET SOMEONE KNOW I WAS THINKING OF THEM
- [ ] PRACTICED BEING MORE PRESENT WITH OTHERS
- [ ] SHARED A STORY
- [ ] WROTE A PERSONAL NOTE OR TEXT

REFLECT

HOW I'D RATE MY FEELING OF CONNECTION TODAY:

| 1 | 2 | 3 | 4 | 5 | 6 | 7 | 8 | 9 | 10 |

LONELY / DISCONNECTED   HIGHLY CONNECTED

THE MOST MEANINGFUL INTERACTION
I HAD TODAY AND HOW IT MADE ME FEEL:

_____
_____
_____
_____
_____
_____
_____
_____

CHALLENGES TO DEVELOPING DEEPER BONDS
AND HOW I CAN OVERCOME THEM:

_____
_____
_____
_____

WAYS I'D LIKE TO CONNECT MORE:

_____
_____
_____
_____
_____

RECORD

DATE ___/___/___

MY GOALS FOR MEANINGFUL CONNECTIONS TODAY:

- [ ] _____
- [ ] _____
- [ ] _____

PEOPLE I'D LIKE TO CONNECT WITH:

_____
_____

WAYS TO STRENGTHEN MY RELATIONSHIPS:

_____
_____

WAYS I CONNECTED WITH OTHERS TODAY:

- [ ] CALLED A FRIEND
- [ ] ENCOURAGED SOMEONE
- [ ] ASKED FOR HELP OR ADVICE
- [ ] PLANNED ONE-ON-ONE TIME
- [ ] PRACTICED ACTIVE LISTENING
- [ ] EXPRESSED MY GRATITUDE TO SOMEONE ELSE
- [ ] SPENT QUALITY TIME WITH A FRIEND OR FAMILY MEMBER
- [ ] HELPED SOMEONE
- [ ] SHARED SOMETHING PERSONAL ABOUT MYSELF
- [ ] PRACTICED VULNERABILITY WITH A TRUSTED FRIEND
- [ ] SHARED A LAUGH
- [ ] TALKED TO SOMEONE NEW
- [ ] COMPLIMENTED SOMEONE
- [ ] COMPLETED A SHARED ACTIVITY
- [ ] NOTED SOMEONE ELSE'S MEANINGFUL DATE, EVENT, OR INTEREST I'D LIKE TO REMEMBER
- [ ] LET SOMEONE KNOW I WAS THINKING OF THEM
- [ ] PRACTICED BEING MORE PRESENT WITH OTHERS
- [ ] SHARED A STORY
- [ ] WROTE A PERSONAL NOTE OR TEXT

REFLECT

HOW I'D RATE MY FEELING OF CONNECTION TODAY:

| 1 | 2 | 3 | 4 | 5 | 6 | 7 | 8 | 9 | 10 |

LONELY / DISCONNECTED   HIGHLY CONNECTED

THE MOST MEANINGFUL INTERACTION
I HAD TODAY AND HOW IT MADE ME FEEL:

_____
_____
_____
_____
_____
_____
_____
_____

CHALLENGES TO DEVELOPING DEEPER BONDS
AND HOW I CAN OVERCOME THEM:

_____
_____
_____
_____

WAYS I'D LIKE TO CONNECT MORE:

_____
_____
_____
_____

RECORD

DATE ___/___/___

MY GOALS FOR MEANINGFUL CONNECTIONS TODAY:

- ☐ _____
- ☐ _____
- ☐ _____

PEOPLE I'D LIKE TO CONNECT WITH:
_____
_____

WAYS TO STRENGTHEN MY RELATIONSHIPS:
_____
_____

WAYS I CONNECTED WITH OTHERS TODAY:

- ☐ CALLED A FRIEND
- ☐ ENCOURAGED SOMEONE
- ☐ ASKED FOR HELP OR ADVICE
- ☐ PLANNED ONE-ON-ONE TIME
- ☐ PRACTICED ACTIVE LISTENING
- ☐ EXPRESSED MY GRATITUDE TO SOMEONE ELSE
- ☐ SPENT QUALITY TIME WITH A FRIEND OR FAMILY MEMBER
- ☐ HELPED SOMEONE
- ☐ SHARED SOMETHING PERSONAL ABOUT MYSELF
- ☐ PRACTICED VULNERABILITY WITH A TRUSTED FRIEND
- ☐ SHARED A LAUGH
- ☐ TALKED TO SOMEONE NEW
- ☐ COMPLIMENTED SOMEONE
- ☐ COMPLETED A SHARED ACTIVITY
- ☐ NOTED SOMEONE ELSE'S MEANINGFUL DATE, EVENT, OR INTEREST I'D LIKE TO REMEMBER
- ☐ LET SOMEONE KNOW I WAS THINKING OF THEM
- ☐ PRACTICED BEING MORE PRESENT WITH OTHERS
- ☐ SHARED A STORY
- ☐ WROTE A PERSONAL NOTE OR TEXT

REFLECT

HOW I'D RATE MY FEELING OF CONNECTION TODAY:

| 1 | 2 | 3 | 4 | 5 | 6 | 7 | 8 | 9 | 10 |

LONELY / DISCONNECTED   HIGHLY CONNECTED

THE MOST MEANINGFUL INTERACTION
I HAD TODAY AND HOW IT MADE ME FEEL:

_____
_____
_____
_____
_____
_____
_____
_____
_____
_____

CHALLENGES TO DEVELOPING DEEPER BONDS
AND HOW I CAN OVERCOME THEM:

_____
_____
_____

WAYS I'D LIKE TO CONNECT MORE:

_____
_____
_____
_____

RECORD

DATE ___/___/___

MY GOALS FOR MEANINGFUL CONNECTIONS TODAY:
- ☐ _____
- ☐ _____
- ☐ _____

PEOPLE I'D LIKE TO CONNECT WITH:
_____
_____

WAYS TO STRENGTHEN MY RELATIONSHIPS:
_____
_____

WAYS I CONNECTED WITH OTHERS TODAY:

- ☐ CALLED A FRIEND
- ☐ ENCOURAGED SOMEONE
- ☐ ASKED FOR HELP OR ADVICE
- ☐ PLANNED ONE-ON-ONE TIME
- ☐ PRACTICED ACTIVE LISTENING
- ☐ EXPRESSED MY GRATITUDE TO SOMEONE ELSE
- ☐ SPENT QUALITY TIME WITH A FRIEND OR FAMILY MEMBER
- ☐ HELPED SOMEONE
- ☐ SHARED SOMETHING PERSONAL ABOUT MYSELF
- ☐ PRACTICED VULNERABILITY WITH A TRUSTED FRIEND
- ☐ SHARED A LAUGH
- ☐ TALKED TO SOMEONE NEW
- ☐ COMPLIMENTED SOMEONE
- ☐ COMPLETED A SHARED ACTIVITY
- ☐ NOTED SOMEONE ELSE'S MEANINGFUL DATE, EVENT, OR INTEREST I'D LIKE TO REMEMBER
- ☐ LET SOMEONE KNOW I WAS THINKING OF THEM
- ☐ PRACTICED BEING MORE PRESENT WITH OTHERS
- ☐ SHARED A STORY
- ☐ WROTE A PERSONAL NOTE OR TEXT

REFLECT

HOW I'D RATE MY FEELING OF CONNECTION TODAY:

| 1 | 2 | 3 | 4 | 5 | 6 | 7 | 8 | 9 | 10 |

LONELY / DISCONNECTED   HIGHLY CONNECTED

THE MOST MEANINGFUL INTERACTION
I HAD TODAY AND HOW IT MADE ME FEEL:

_____
_____
_____
_____
_____
_____
_____
_____
_____

CHALLENGES TO DEVELOPING DEEPER BONDS
AND HOW I CAN OVERCOME THEM:

_____
_____
_____

WAYS I'D LIKE TO CONNECT MORE:

_____
_____
_____
_____

RECORD

DATE ___/___/___

MY GOALS FOR MEANINGFUL CONNECTIONS TODAY:

- ☐ _____
- ☐ _____
- ☐ _____

PEOPLE I'D LIKE TO CONNECT WITH:

_____
_____

WAYS TO STRENGTHEN MY RELATIONSHIPS:

_____
_____

WAYS I CONNECTED WITH OTHERS TODAY:

- ☐ CALLED A FRIEND
- ☐ ENCOURAGED SOMEONE
- ☐ ASKED FOR HELP OR ADVICE
- ☐ PLANNED ONE-ON-ONE TIME
- ☐ PRACTICED ACTIVE LISTENING
- ☐ EXPRESSED MY GRATITUDE TO SOMEONE ELSE
- ☐ SPENT QUALITY TIME WITH A FRIEND OR FAMILY MEMBER
- ☐ HELPED SOMEONE
- ☐ SHARED SOMETHING PERSONAL ABOUT MYSELF
- ☐ PRACTICED VULNERABILITY WITH A TRUSTED FRIEND
- ☐ SHARED A LAUGH
- ☐ TALKED TO SOMEONE NEW
- ☐ COMPLIMENTED SOMEONE
- ☐ COMPLETED A SHARED ACTIVITY
- ☐ NOTED SOMEONE ELSE'S MEANINGFUL DATE, EVENT, OR INTEREST I'D LIKE TO REMEMBER
- ☐ LET SOMEONE KNOW I WAS THINKING OF THEM
- ☐ PRACTICED BEING MORE PRESENT WITH OTHERS
- ☐ SHARED A STORY
- ☐ WROTE A PERSONAL NOTE OR TEXT

REFLECT

HOW I'D RATE MY FEELING OF CONNECTION TODAY:

| 1 | 2 | 3 | 4 | 5 | 6 | 7 | 8 | 9 | 10 |

LONELY / DISCONNECTED   HIGHLY CONNECTED

THE MOST MEANINGFUL INTERACTION
I HAD TODAY AND HOW IT MADE ME FEEL:

___

CHALLENGES TO DEVELOPING DEEPER BONDS
AND HOW I CAN OVERCOME THEM:

___

WAYS I'D LIKE TO CONNECT MORE:

___

RECORD

DATE ____/____/____

MY GOALS FOR MEANINGFUL CONNECTIONS TODAY:

- [ ] _____
- [ ] _____
- [ ] _____

PEOPLE I'D LIKE TO CONNECT WITH:

_____
_____

WAYS TO STRENGTHEN MY RELATIONSHIPS:

_____
_____

WAYS I CONNECTED WITH OTHERS TODAY:

- [ ] CALLED A FRIEND
- [ ] ENCOURAGED SOMEONE
- [ ] ASKED FOR HELP OR ADVICE
- [ ] PLANNED ONE-ON-ONE TIME
- [ ] PRACTICED ACTIVE LISTENING
- [ ] EXPRESSED MY GRATITUDE TO SOMEONE ELSE
- [ ] SPENT QUALITY TIME WITH A FRIEND OR FAMILY MEMBER
- [ ] HELPED SOMEONE
- [ ] SHARED SOMETHING PERSONAL ABOUT MYSELF
- [ ] PRACTICED VULNERABILITY WITH A TRUSTED FRIEND
- [ ] SHARED A LAUGH
- [ ] TALKED TO SOMEONE NEW
- [ ] COMPLIMENTED SOMEONE
- [ ] COMPLETED A SHARED ACTIVITY
- [ ] NOTED SOMEONE ELSE'S MEANINGFUL DATE, EVENT, OR INTEREST I'D LIKE TO REMEMBER
- [ ] LET SOMEONE KNOW I WAS THINKING OF THEM
- [ ] PRACTICED BEING MORE PRESENT WITH OTHERS
- [ ] SHARED A STORY
- [ ] WROTE A PERSONAL NOTE OR TEXT

REFLECT

HOW I'D RATE MY FEELING OF CONNECTION TODAY:

| 1 | 2 | 3 | 4 | 5 | 6 | 7 | 8 | 9 | 10 |

LONELY / DISCONNECTED   HIGHLY CONNECTED

THE MOST MEANINGFUL INTERACTION I HAD TODAY AND HOW IT MADE ME FEEL:

_____
_____
_____
_____
_____
_____
_____
_____
_____

CHALLENGES TO DEVELOPING DEEPER BONDS AND HOW I CAN OVERCOME THEM:

_____
_____
_____

WAYS I'D LIKE TO CONNECT MORE:

_____
_____
_____
_____

RECORD

DATE ___/___/___

MY GOALS FOR MEANINGFUL CONNECTIONS TODAY:

- [ ] _____
- [ ] _____
- [ ] _____

PEOPLE I'D LIKE TO CONNECT WITH:

_____
_____

WAYS TO STRENGTHEN MY RELATIONSHIPS:

_____
_____

WAYS I CONNECTED WITH OTHERS TODAY:

- [ ] CALLED A FRIEND
- [ ] ENCOURAGED SOMEONE
- [ ] ASKED FOR HELP OR ADVICE
- [ ] PLANNED ONE-ON-ONE TIME
- [ ] PRACTICED ACTIVE LISTENING
- [ ] EXPRESSED MY GRATITUDE TO SOMEONE ELSE
- [ ] SPENT QUALITY TIME WITH A FRIEND OR FAMILY MEMBER
- [ ] HELPED SOMEONE
- [ ] SHARED SOMETHING PERSONAL ABOUT MYSELF
- [ ] PRACTICED VULNERABILITY WITH A TRUSTED FRIEND
- [ ] SHARED A LAUGH
- [ ] TALKED TO SOMEONE NEW
- [ ] COMPLIMENTED SOMEONE
- [ ] COMPLETED A SHARED ACTIVITY
- [ ] NOTED SOMEONE ELSE'S MEANINGFUL DATE, EVENT, OR INTEREST I'D LIKE TO REMEMBER
- [ ] LET SOMEONE KNOW I WAS THINKING OF THEM
- [ ] PRACTICED BEING MORE PRESENT WITH OTHERS
- [ ] SHARED A STORY
- [ ] WROTE A PERSONAL NOTE OR TEXT

REFLECT

HOW I'D RATE MY FEELING OF CONNECTION TODAY:

| 1 | 2 | 3 | 4 | 5 | 6 | 7 | 8 | 9 | 10 |

LONELY / DISCONNECTEDHIGHLY CONNECTED

THE MOST MEANINGFUL INTERACTION
I HAD TODAY AND HOW IT MADE ME FEEL:

_____
_____
_____
_____
_____
_____
_____
_____

CHALLENGES TO DEVELOPING DEEPER BONDS
AND HOW I CAN OVERCOME THEM:

_____
_____
_____

WAYS I'D LIKE TO CONNECT MORE:

_____
_____
_____
_____

RECORD

DATE ___/___/___

MY GOALS FOR MEANINGFUL CONNECTIONS TODAY:

- ☐ _____
- ☐ _____
- ☐ _____

PEOPLE I'D LIKE TO CONNECT WITH:

_____
_____

WAYS TO STRENGTHEN MY RELATIONSHIPS:

_____
_____

WAYS I CONNECTED WITH OTHERS TODAY:

- ☐ CALLED A FRIEND
- ☐ ENCOURAGED SOMEONE
- ☐ ASKED FOR HELP OR ADVICE
- ☐ PLANNED ONE-ON-ONE TIME
- ☐ PRACTICED ACTIVE LISTENING
- ☐ EXPRESSED MY GRATITUDE TO SOMEONE ELSE
- ☐ SPENT QUALITY TIME WITH A FRIEND OR FAMILY MEMBER
- ☐ HELPED SOMEONE
- ☐ SHARED SOMETHING PERSONAL ABOUT MYSELF
- ☐ PRACTICED VULNERABILITY WITH A TRUSTED FRIEND
- ☐ SHARED A LAUGH
- ☐ TALKED TO SOMEONE NEW
- ☐ COMPLIMENTED SOMEONE
- ☐ COMPLETED A SHARED ACTIVITY
- ☐ NOTED SOMEONE ELSE'S MEANINGFUL DATE, EVENT, OR INTEREST I'D LIKE TO REMEMBER
- ☐ LET SOMEONE KNOW I WAS THINKING OF THEM
- ☐ PRACTICED BEING MORE PRESENT WITH OTHERS
- ☐ SHARED A STORY
- ☐ WROTE A PERSONAL NOTE OR TEXT

REFLECT

HOW I'D RATE MY FEELING OF CONNECTION TODAY:

| 1 | 2 | 3 | 4 | 5 | 6 | 7 | 8 | 9 | 10 |

LONELY / DISCONNECTED   HIGHLY CONNECTED

THE MOST MEANINGFUL INTERACTION
I HAD TODAY AND HOW IT MADE ME FEEL:

_____
_____
_____
_____
_____
_____
_____
_____
_____

CHALLENGES TO DEVELOPING DEEPER BONDS
AND HOW I CAN OVERCOME THEM:

_____
_____
_____

WAYS I'D LIKE TO CONNECT MORE:

_____
_____
_____
_____
_____

RECORD

DATE ___/___/___

MY GOALS FOR MEANINGFUL CONNECTIONS TODAY:

- ☐ _____
- ☐ _____
- ☐ _____

PEOPLE I'D LIKE TO CONNECT WITH:

_____
_____

WAYS TO STRENGTHEN MY RELATIONSHIPS:

_____
_____

WAYS I CONNECTED WITH OTHERS TODAY:

- ☐ CALLED A FRIEND
- ☐ ENCOURAGED SOMEONE
- ☐ ASKED FOR HELP OR ADVICE
- ☐ PLANNED ONE-ON-ONE TIME
- ☐ PRACTICED ACTIVE LISTENING
- ☐ EXPRESSED MY GRATITUDE TO SOMEONE ELSE
- ☐ SPENT QUALITY TIME WITH A FRIEND OR FAMILY MEMBER
- ☐ HELPED SOMEONE
- ☐ SHARED SOMETHING PERSONAL ABOUT MYSELF
- ☐ PRACTICED VULNERABILITY WITH A TRUSTED FRIEND
- ☐ SHARED A LAUGH
- ☐ TALKED TO SOMEONE NEW
- ☐ COMPLIMENTED SOMEONE
- ☐ COMPLETED A SHARED ACTIVITY
- ☐ NOTED SOMEONE ELSE'S MEANINGFUL DATE, EVENT, OR INTEREST I'D LIKE TO REMEMBER
- ☐ LET SOMEONE KNOW I WAS THINKING OF THEM
- ☐ PRACTICED BEING MORE PRESENT WITH OTHERS
- ☐ SHARED A STORY
- ☐ WROTE A PERSONAL NOTE OR TEXT

REFLECT

HOW I'D RATE MY FEELING OF CONNECTION TODAY:

| 1 | 2 | 3 | 4 | 5 | 6 | 7 | 8 | 9 | 10 |

LONELY / DISCONNECTED   HIGHLY CONNECTED

THE MOST MEANINGFUL INTERACTION
I HAD TODAY AND HOW IT MADE ME FEEL:

_____
_____
_____
_____
_____
_____
_____
_____
_____

CHALLENGES TO DEVELOPING DEEPER BONDS
AND HOW I CAN OVERCOME THEM:

_____
_____
_____

WAYS I'D LIKE TO CONNECT MORE:

_____
_____
_____
_____

RECORD

DATE ___/___/___

MY GOALS FOR MEANINGFUL CONNECTIONS TODAY:
- ☐ _____
- ☐ _____
- ☐ _____

PEOPLE I'D LIKE TO CONNECT WITH:
_____
_____

WAYS TO STRENGTHEN MY RELATIONSHIPS:
_____
_____

WAYS I CONNECTED WITH OTHERS TODAY:

- ☐ CALLED A FRIEND
- ☐ ENCOURAGED SOMEONE
- ☐ ASKED FOR HELP OR ADVICE
- ☐ PLANNED ONE-ON-ONE TIME
- ☐ PRACTICED ACTIVE LISTENING
- ☐ EXPRESSED MY GRATITUDE TO SOMEONE ELSE
- ☐ SPENT QUALITY TIME WITH A FRIEND OR FAMILY MEMBER
- ☐ HELPED SOMEONE
- ☐ SHARED SOMETHING PERSONAL ABOUT MYSELF
- ☐ PRACTICED VULNERABILITY WITH A TRUSTED FRIEND
- ☐ SHARED A LAUGH
- ☐ TALKED TO SOMEONE NEW
- ☐ COMPLIMENTED SOMEONE
- ☐ COMPLETED A SHARED ACTIVITY
- ☐ NOTED SOMEONE ELSE'S MEANINGFUL DATE, EVENT, OR INTEREST I'D LIKE TO REMEMBER
- ☐ LET SOMEONE KNOW I WAS THINKING OF THEM
- ☐ PRACTICED BEING MORE PRESENT WITH OTHERS
- ☐ SHARED A STORY
- ☐ WROTE A PERSONAL NOTE OR TEXT

REFLECT

HOW I'D RATE MY FEELING OF CONNECTION TODAY:

| 1 | 2 | 3 | 4 | 5 | 6 | 7 | 8 | 9 | 10 |

LONELY / DISCONNECTED   HIGHLY CONNECTED

THE MOST MEANINGFUL INTERACTION
I HAD TODAY AND HOW IT MADE ME FEEL:

_____
_____
_____
_____
_____
_____
_____
_____
_____

CHALLENGES TO DEVELOPING DEEPER BONDS
AND HOW I CAN OVERCOME THEM:

_____
_____
_____

WAYS I'D LIKE TO CONNECT MORE:

_____
_____
_____
_____

RECORD

DATE ___/___/___

MY GOALS FOR MEANINGFUL CONNECTIONS TODAY:

☐ _____
☐ _____
☐ _____

PEOPLE I'D LIKE TO CONNECT WITH:

_____
_____

WAYS TO STRENGTHEN MY RELATIONSHIPS:

_____
_____

WAYS I CONNECTED WITH OTHERS TODAY:

☐ CALLED A FRIEND
☐ ENCOURAGED SOMEONE
☐ ASKED FOR HELP OR ADVICE
☐ PLANNED ONE-ON-ONE TIME
☐ PRACTICED ACTIVE LISTENING
☐ EXPRESSED MY GRATITUDE TO SOMEONE ELSE
☐ SPENT QUALITY TIME WITH A FRIEND OR FAMILY MEMBER
☐ HELPED SOMEONE
☐ SHARED SOMETHING PERSONAL ABOUT MYSELF
☐ PRACTICED VULNERABILITY WITH A TRUSTED FRIEND

☐ SHARED A LAUGH
☐ TALKED TO SOMEONE NEW
☐ COMPLIMENTED SOMEONE
☐ COMPLETED A SHARED ACTIVITY
☐ NOTED SOMEONE ELSE'S MEANINGFUL DATE, EVENT, OR INTEREST I'D LIKE TO REMEMBER
☐ LET SOMEONE KNOW I WAS THINKING OF THEM
☐ PRACTICED BEING MORE PRESENT WITH OTHERS
☐ SHARED A STORY
☐ WROTE A PERSONAL NOTE OR TEXT

REFLECT

HOW I'D RATE MY FEELING OF CONNECTION TODAY:

| 1 | 2 | 3 | 4 | 5 | 6 | 7 | 8 | 9 | 10 |

LONELY / DISCONNECTED   HIGHLY CONNECTED

THE MOST MEANINGFUL INTERACTION
I HAD TODAY AND HOW IT MADE ME FEEL:

_____
_____
_____
_____
_____
_____
_____
_____
_____

CHALLENGES TO DEVELOPING DEEPER BONDS
AND HOW I CAN OVERCOME THEM:

_____
_____
_____

WAYS I'D LIKE TO CONNECT MORE:

_____
_____
_____
_____

RECORD

DATE ___/___/___

MY GOALS FOR MEANINGFUL CONNECTIONS TODAY:
- ☐ _____
- ☐ _____
- ☐ _____

PEOPLE I'D LIKE TO CONNECT WITH:
_____
_____

WAYS TO STRENGTHEN MY RELATIONSHIPS:
_____
_____

WAYS I CONNECTED WITH OTHERS TODAY:

- ☐ CALLED A FRIEND
- ☐ ENCOURAGED SOMEONE
- ☐ ASKED FOR HELP OR ADVICE
- ☐ PLANNED ONE-ON-ONE TIME
- ☐ PRACTICED ACTIVE LISTENING
- ☐ EXPRESSED MY GRATITUDE TO SOMEONE ELSE
- ☐ SPENT QUALITY TIME WITH A FRIEND OR FAMILY MEMBER
- ☐ HELPED SOMEONE
- ☐ SHARED SOMETHING PERSONAL ABOUT MYSELF
- ☐ PRACTICED VULNERABILITY WITH A TRUSTED FRIEND
- ☐ SHARED A LAUGH
- ☐ TALKED TO SOMEONE NEW
- ☐ COMPLIMENTED SOMEONE
- ☐ COMPLETED A SHARED ACTIVITY
- ☐ NOTED SOMEONE ELSE'S MEANINGFUL DATE, EVENT, OR INTEREST I'D LIKE TO REMEMBER
- ☐ LET SOMEONE KNOW I WAS THINKING OF THEM
- ☐ PRACTICED BEING MORE PRESENT WITH OTHERS
- ☐ SHARED A STORY
- ☐ WROTE A PERSONAL NOTE OR TEXT

REFLECT

HOW I'D RATE MY FEELING OF CONNECTION TODAY:

| 1 | 2 | 3 | 4 | 5 | 6 | 7 | 8 | 9 | 10 |

LONELY / DISCONNECTED   HIGHLY CONNECTED

THE MOST MEANINGFUL INTERACTION
I HAD TODAY AND HOW IT MADE ME FEEL:

_____
_____
_____
_____
_____
_____
_____
_____

CHALLENGES TO DEVELOPING DEEPER BONDS
AND HOW I CAN OVERCOME THEM:

_____
_____
_____

WAYS I'D LIKE TO CONNECT MORE:

_____
_____
_____
_____

RECORD

DATE ___/___/___

MY GOALS FOR MEANINGFUL CONNECTIONS TODAY:

- ☐ _____
- ☐ _____
- ☐ _____

PEOPLE I'D LIKE TO CONNECT WITH:

_____
_____

WAYS TO STRENGTHEN MY RELATIONSHIPS:

_____
_____

WAYS I CONNECTED WITH OTHERS TODAY:

- ☐ CALLED A FRIEND
- ☐ ENCOURAGED SOMEONE
- ☐ ASKED FOR HELP OR ADVICE
- ☐ PLANNED ONE-ON-ONE TIME
- ☐ PRACTICED ACTIVE LISTENING
- ☐ EXPRESSED MY GRATITUDE TO SOMEONE ELSE
- ☐ SPENT QUALITY TIME WITH A FRIEND OR FAMILY MEMBER
- ☐ HELPED SOMEONE
- ☐ SHARED SOMETHING PERSONAL ABOUT MYSELF
- ☐ PRACTICED VULNERABILITY WITH A TRUSTED FRIEND
- ☐ SHARED A LAUGH
- ☐ TALKED TO SOMEONE NEW
- ☐ COMPLIMENTED SOMEONE
- ☐ COMPLETED A SHARED ACTIVITY
- ☐ NOTED SOMEONE ELSE'S MEANINGFUL DATE, EVENT, OR INTEREST I'D LIKE TO REMEMBER
- ☐ LET SOMEONE KNOW I WAS THINKING OF THEM
- ☐ PRACTICED BEING MORE PRESENT WITH OTHERS
- ☐ SHARED A STORY
- ☐ WROTE A PERSONAL NOTE OR TEXT

REFLECT

HOW I'D RATE MY FEELING OF CONNECTION TODAY:

| 1 | 2 | 3 | 4 | 5 | 6 | 7 | 8 | 9 | 10 |

LONELY / DISCONNECTED   HIGHLY CONNECTED

THE MOST MEANINGFUL INTERACTION
I HAD TODAY AND HOW IT MADE ME FEEL:

_____
_____
_____
_____
_____
_____
_____
_____
_____

CHALLENGES TO DEVELOPING DEEPER BONDS
AND HOW I CAN OVERCOME THEM:

_____
_____
_____

WAYS I'D LIKE TO CONNECT MORE:

_____
_____
_____
_____
_____

RECORD

DATE ___/___/___

MY GOALS FOR MEANINGFUL CONNECTIONS TODAY:

- [ ] _____
- [ ] _____
- [ ] _____

PEOPLE I'D LIKE TO CONNECT WITH:

_____
_____

WAYS TO STRENGTHEN MY RELATIONSHIPS:

_____
_____

WAYS I CONNECTED WITH OTHERS TODAY:

- [ ] CALLED A FRIEND
- [ ] ENCOURAGED SOMEONE
- [ ] ASKED FOR HELP OR ADVICE
- [ ] PLANNED ONE-ON-ONE TIME
- [ ] PRACTICED ACTIVE LISTENING
- [ ] EXPRESSED MY GRATITUDE TO SOMEONE ELSE
- [ ] SPENT QUALITY TIME WITH A FRIEND OR FAMILY MEMBER
- [ ] HELPED SOMEONE
- [ ] SHARED SOMETHING PERSONAL ABOUT MYSELF
- [ ] PRACTICED VULNERABILITY WITH A TRUSTED FRIEND
- [ ] SHARED A LAUGH
- [ ] TALKED TO SOMEONE NEW
- [ ] COMPLIMENTED SOMEONE
- [ ] COMPLETED A SHARED ACTIVITY
- [ ] NOTED SOMEONE ELSE'S MEANINGFUL DATE, EVENT, OR INTEREST I'D LIKE TO REMEMBER
- [ ] LET SOMEONE KNOW I WAS THINKING OF THEM
- [ ] PRACTICED BEING MORE PRESENT WITH OTHERS
- [ ] SHARED A STORY
- [ ] WROTE A PERSONAL NOTE OR TEXT

REFLECT

HOW I'D RATE MY FEELING OF CONNECTION TODAY:

| 1 | 2 | 3 | 4 | 5 | 6 | 7 | 8 | 9 | 10 |

LONELY / DISCONNECTED   HIGHLY CONNECTED

THE MOST MEANINGFUL INTERACTION
I HAD TODAY AND HOW IT MADE ME FEEL:

_____
_____
_____
_____
_____
_____
_____
_____
_____

CHALLENGES TO DEVELOPING DEEPER BONDS
AND HOW I CAN OVERCOME THEM:

_____
_____
_____

WAYS I'D LIKE TO CONNECT MORE:

_____
_____
_____
_____

RECORD

DATE ___/___/___

MY GOALS FOR MEANINGFUL CONNECTIONS TODAY:

- [ ] _____
- [ ] _____
- [ ] _____

PEOPLE I'D LIKE TO CONNECT WITH:

_____

_____

WAYS TO STRENGTHEN MY RELATIONSHIPS:

_____

_____

WAYS I CONNECTED WITH OTHERS TODAY:

- [ ] CALLED A FRIEND
- [ ] ENCOURAGED SOMEONE
- [ ] ASKED FOR HELP OR ADVICE
- [ ] PLANNED ONE-ON-ONE TIME
- [ ] PRACTICED ACTIVE LISTENING
- [ ] EXPRESSED MY GRATITUDE TO SOMEONE ELSE
- [ ] SPENT QUALITY TIME WITH A FRIEND OR FAMILY MEMBER
- [ ] HELPED SOMEONE
- [ ] SHARED SOMETHING PERSONAL ABOUT MYSELF
- [ ] PRACTICED VULNERABILITY WITH A TRUSTED FRIEND
- [ ] SHARED A LAUGH
- [ ] TALKED TO SOMEONE NEW
- [ ] COMPLIMENTED SOMEONE
- [ ] COMPLETED A SHARED ACTIVITY
- [ ] NOTED SOMEONE ELSE'S MEANINGFUL DATE, EVENT, OR INTEREST I'D LIKE TO REMEMBER
- [ ] LET SOMEONE KNOW I WAS THINKING OF THEM
- [ ] PRACTICED BEING MORE PRESENT WITH OTHERS
- [ ] SHARED A STORY
- [ ] WROTE A PERSONAL NOTE OR TEXT

REFLECT

HOW I'D RATE MY FEELING OF CONNECTION TODAY:

| 1 | 2 | 3 | 4 | 5 | 6 | 7 | 8 | 9 | 10 |

LONELY / DISCONNECTED　　　　　　　　　　　　　　　　　HIGHLY CONNECTED

THE MOST MEANINGFUL INTERACTION
I HAD TODAY AND HOW IT MADE ME FEEL:

_____
_____
_____
_____
_____
_____
_____
_____
_____
_____

CHALLENGES TO DEVELOPING DEEPER BONDS
AND HOW I CAN OVERCOME THEM:

_____
_____
_____

WAYS I'D LIKE TO CONNECT MORE:

_____
_____
_____
_____

RECORD

DATE ___/___/___

MY GOALS FOR MEANINGFUL CONNECTIONS TODAY:

- ☐ _____
- ☐ _____
- ☐ _____

PEOPLE I'D LIKE TO CONNECT WITH:

_____
_____

WAYS TO STRENGTHEN MY RELATIONSHIPS:

_____
_____

WAYS I CONNECTED WITH OTHERS TODAY:

- ☐ CALLED A FRIEND
- ☐ ENCOURAGED SOMEONE
- ☐ ASKED FOR HELP OR ADVICE
- ☐ PLANNED ONE-ON-ONE TIME
- ☐ PRACTICED ACTIVE LISTENING
- ☐ EXPRESSED MY GRATITUDE TO SOMEONE ELSE
- ☐ SPENT QUALITY TIME WITH A FRIEND OR FAMILY MEMBER
- ☐ HELPED SOMEONE
- ☐ SHARED SOMETHING PERSONAL ABOUT MYSELF
- ☐ PRACTICED VULNERABILITY WITH A TRUSTED FRIEND
- ☐ SHARED A LAUGH
- ☐ TALKED TO SOMEONE NEW
- ☐ COMPLIMENTED SOMEONE
- ☐ COMPLETED A SHARED ACTIVITY
- ☐ NOTED SOMEONE ELSE'S MEANINGFUL DATE, EVENT, OR INTEREST I'D LIKE TO REMEMBER
- ☐ LET SOMEONE KNOW I WAS THINKING OF THEM
- ☐ PRACTICED BEING MORE PRESENT WITH OTHERS
- ☐ SHARED A STORY
- ☐ WROTE A PERSONAL NOTE OR TEXT

REFLECT

HOW I'D RATE MY FEELING OF CONNECTION TODAY:

| 1 | 2 | 3 | 4 | 5 | 6 | 7 | 8 | 9 | 10 |

LONELY / DISCONNECTED　　　　　　　　　　　　　　　　HIGHLY CONNECTED

THE MOST MEANINGFUL INTERACTION
I HAD TODAY AND HOW IT MADE ME FEEL:

_____
_____
_____
_____
_____
_____
_____
_____
_____

CHALLENGES TO DEVELOPING DEEPER BONDS
AND HOW I CAN OVERCOME THEM:

_____
_____
_____

WAYS I'D LIKE TO CONNECT MORE:

_____
_____
_____
_____

RECORD

DATE ___/___/___

MY GOALS FOR MEANINGFUL CONNECTIONS TODAY:
- [ ] _____
- [ ] _____
- [ ] _____

PEOPLE I'D LIKE TO CONNECT WITH:
_____
_____

WAYS TO STRENGTHEN MY RELATIONSHIPS:
_____
_____

WAYS I CONNECTED WITH OTHERS TODAY:

- [ ] CALLED A FRIEND
- [ ] ENCOURAGED SOMEONE
- [ ] ASKED FOR HELP OR ADVICE
- [ ] PLANNED ONE-ON-ONE TIME
- [ ] PRACTICED ACTIVE LISTENING
- [ ] EXPRESSED MY GRATITUDE TO SOMEONE ELSE
- [ ] SPENT QUALITY TIME WITH A FRIEND OR FAMILY MEMBER
- [ ] HELPED SOMEONE
- [ ] SHARED SOMETHING PERSONAL ABOUT MYSELF
- [ ] PRACTICED VULNERABILITY WITH A TRUSTED FRIEND
- [ ] SHARED A LAUGH
- [ ] TALKED TO SOMEONE NEW
- [ ] COMPLIMENTED SOMEONE
- [ ] COMPLETED A SHARED ACTIVITY
- [ ] NOTED SOMEONE ELSE'S MEANINGFUL DATE, EVENT, OR INTEREST I'D LIKE TO REMEMBER
- [ ] LET SOMEONE KNOW I WAS THINKING OF THEM
- [ ] PRACTICED BEING MORE PRESENT WITH OTHERS
- [ ] SHARED A STORY
- [ ] WROTE A PERSONAL NOTE OR TEXT

REFLECT

HOW I'D RATE MY FEELING OF CONNECTION TODAY:

| 1 | 2 | 3 | 4 | 5 | 6 | 7 | 8 | 9 | 10 |

LONELY / DISCONNECTED   HIGHLY CONNECTED

THE MOST MEANINGFUL INTERACTION
I HAD TODAY AND HOW IT MADE ME FEEL:
_____
_____
_____
_____
_____
_____
_____
_____

CHALLENGES TO DEVELOPING DEEPER BONDS
AND HOW I CAN OVERCOME THEM:
_____
_____
_____

WAYS I'D LIKE TO CONNECT MORE:
_____
_____
_____
_____

RECORD

DATE ___/___/___

MY GOALS FOR MEANINGFUL CONNECTIONS TODAY:

- ☐ _____
- ☐ _____
- ☐ _____

PEOPLE I'D LIKE TO CONNECT WITH:

_____
_____

WAYS TO STRENGTHEN MY RELATIONSHIPS:

_____
_____

WAYS I CONNECTED WITH OTHERS TODAY:

- ☐ CALLED A FRIEND
- ☐ ENCOURAGED SOMEONE
- ☐ ASKED FOR HELP OR ADVICE
- ☐ PLANNED ONE-ON-ONE TIME
- ☐ PRACTICED ACTIVE LISTENING
- ☐ EXPRESSED MY GRATITUDE TO SOMEONE ELSE
- ☐ SPENT QUALITY TIME WITH A FRIEND OR FAMILY MEMBER
- ☐ HELPED SOMEONE
- ☐ SHARED SOMETHING PERSONAL ABOUT MYSELF
- ☐ PRACTICED VULNERABILITY WITH A TRUSTED FRIEND
- ☐ SHARED A LAUGH
- ☐ TALKED TO SOMEONE NEW
- ☐ COMPLIMENTED SOMEONE
- ☐ COMPLETED A SHARED ACTIVITY
- ☐ NOTED SOMEONE ELSE'S MEANINGFUL DATE, EVENT, OR INTEREST I'D LIKE TO REMEMBER
- ☐ LET SOMEONE KNOW I WAS THINKING OF THEM
- ☐ PRACTICED BEING MORE PRESENT WITH OTHERS
- ☐ SHARED A STORY
- ☐ WROTE A PERSONAL NOTE OR TEXT

REFLECT

HOW I'D RATE MY FEELING OF CONNECTION TODAY:

| 1 | 2 | 3 | 4 | 5 | 6 | 7 | 8 | 9 | 10 |

LONELY / DISCONNECTED   HIGHLY CONNECTED

THE MOST MEANINGFUL INTERACTION
I HAD TODAY AND HOW IT MADE ME FEEL:

_____
_____
_____
_____
_____
_____
_____
_____

CHALLENGES TO DEVELOPING DEEPER BONDS
AND HOW I CAN OVERCOME THEM:

_____
_____
_____

WAYS I'D LIKE TO CONNECT MORE:

_____
_____
_____
_____

RECORD

DATE ___/___/___

MY GOALS FOR MEANINGFUL CONNECTIONS TODAY:
- ☐ _____
- ☐ _____
- ☐ _____

PEOPLE I'D LIKE TO CONNECT WITH:
_____

WAYS TO STRENGTHEN MY RELATIONSHIPS:
_____
_____

WAYS I CONNECTED WITH OTHERS TODAY:

- ☐ CALLED A FRIEND
- ☐ ENCOURAGED SOMEONE
- ☐ ASKED FOR HELP OR ADVICE
- ☐ PLANNED ONE-ON-ONE TIME
- ☐ PRACTICED ACTIVE LISTENING
- ☐ EXPRESSED MY GRATITUDE TO SOMEONE ELSE
- ☐ SPENT QUALITY TIME WITH A FRIEND OR FAMILY MEMBER
- ☐ HELPED SOMEONE
- ☐ SHARED SOMETHING PERSONAL ABOUT MYSELF
- ☐ PRACTICED VULNERABILITY WITH A TRUSTED FRIEND
- ☐ SHARED A LAUGH
- ☐ TALKED TO SOMEONE NEW
- ☐ COMPLIMENTED SOMEONE
- ☐ COMPLETED A SHARED ACTIVITY
- ☐ NOTED SOMEONE ELSE'S MEANINGFUL DATE, EVENT, OR INTEREST I'D LIKE TO REMEMBER
- ☐ LET SOMEONE KNOW I WAS THINKING OF THEM
- ☐ PRACTICED BEING MORE PRESENT WITH OTHERS
- ☐ SHARED A STORY
- ☐ WROTE A PERSONAL NOTE OR TEXT

REFLECT

HOW I'D RATE MY FEELING OF CONNECTION TODAY:

| 1 | 2 | 3 | 4 | 5 | 6 | 7 | 8 | 9 | 10 |

LONELY / DISCONNECTED   HIGHLY CONNECTED

THE MOST MEANINGFUL INTERACTION
I HAD TODAY AND HOW IT MADE ME FEEL:
_____
_____
_____
_____
_____
_____
_____
_____

CHALLENGES TO DEVELOPING DEEPER BONDS
AND HOW I CAN OVERCOME THEM:
_____
_____
_____
_____

WAYS I'D LIKE TO CONNECT MORE:
_____
_____
_____
_____

RECORD

DATE ___/___/___

MY GOALS FOR MEANINGFUL CONNECTIONS TODAY:
- ☐ _____
- ☐ _____
- ☐ _____

PEOPLE I'D LIKE TO CONNECT WITH:
_____
_____

WAYS TO STRENGTHEN MY RELATIONSHIPS:
_____
_____

WAYS I CONNECTED WITH OTHERS TODAY:

- ☐ CALLED A FRIEND
- ☐ ENCOURAGED SOMEONE
- ☐ ASKED FOR HELP OR ADVICE
- ☐ PLANNED ONE-ON-ONE TIME
- ☐ PRACTICED ACTIVE LISTENING
- ☐ EXPRESSED MY GRATITUDE TO SOMEONE ELSE
- ☐ SPENT QUALITY TIME WITH A FRIEND OR FAMILY MEMBER
- ☐ HELPED SOMEONE
- ☐ SHARED SOMETHING PERSONAL ABOUT MYSELF
- ☐ PRACTICED VULNERABILITY WITH A TRUSTED FRIEND
- ☐ SHARED A LAUGH
- ☐ TALKED TO SOMEONE NEW
- ☐ COMPLIMENTED SOMEONE
- ☐ COMPLETED A SHARED ACTIVITY
- ☐ NOTED SOMEONE ELSE'S MEANINGFUL DATE, EVENT, OR INTEREST I'D LIKE TO REMEMBER
- ☐ LET SOMEONE KNOW I WAS THINKING OF THEM
- ☐ PRACTICED BEING MORE PRESENT WITH OTHERS
- ☐ SHARED A STORY
- ☐ WROTE A PERSONAL NOTE OR TEXT

REFLECT

HOW I'D RATE MY FEELING OF CONNECTION TODAY:

| 1 | 2 | 3 | 4 | 5 | 6 | 7 | 8 | 9 | 10 |

LONELY / DISCONNECTED   HIGHLY CONNECTED

THE MOST MEANINGFUL INTERACTION
I HAD TODAY AND HOW IT MADE ME FEEL:

_____
_____
_____
_____
_____
_____
_____

CHALLENGES TO DEVELOPING DEEPER BONDS
AND HOW I CAN OVERCOME THEM:

_____
_____
_____
_____

WAYS I'D LIKE TO CONNECT MORE:

_____
_____
_____
_____

RECORD

DATE ___/___/___

MY GOALS FOR MEANINGFUL CONNECTIONS TODAY:

☐ _____
☐ _____
☐ _____

PEOPLE I'D LIKE TO CONNECT WITH:

_____
_____

WAYS TO STRENGTHEN MY RELATIONSHIPS:

_____
_____

WAYS I CONNECTED WITH OTHERS TODAY:

- ☐ CALLED A FRIEND
- ☐ ENCOURAGED SOMEONE
- ☐ ASKED FOR HELP OR ADVICE
- ☐ PLANNED ONE-ON-ONE TIME
- ☐ PRACTICED ACTIVE LISTENING
- ☐ EXPRESSED MY GRATITUDE TO SOMEONE ELSE
- ☐ SPENT QUALITY TIME WITH A FRIEND OR FAMILY MEMBER
- ☐ HELPED SOMEONE
- ☐ SHARED SOMETHING PERSONAL ABOUT MYSELF
- ☐ PRACTICED VULNERABILITY WITH A TRUSTED FRIEND
- ☐ SHARED A LAUGH
- ☐ TALKED TO SOMEONE NEW
- ☐ COMPLIMENTED SOMEONE
- ☐ COMPLETED A SHARED ACTIVITY
- ☐ NOTED SOMEONE ELSE'S MEANINGFUL DATE, EVENT, OR INTEREST I'D LIKE TO REMEMBER
- ☐ LET SOMEONE KNOW I WAS THINKING OF THEM
- ☐ PRACTICED BEING MORE PRESENT WITH OTHERS
- ☐ SHARED A STORY
- ☐ WROTE A PERSONAL NOTE OR TEXT

REFLECT

HOW I'D RATE MY FEELING OF CONNECTION TODAY:

| 1 | 2 | 3 | 4 | 5 | 6 | 7 | 8 | 9 | 10 |

LONELY / DISCONNECTEDHIGHLY CONNECTED

THE MOST MEANINGFUL INTERACTION
I HAD TODAY AND HOW IT MADE ME FEEL:
_____
_____
_____
_____
_____
_____
_____
_____
_____

CHALLENGES TO DEVELOPING DEEPER BONDS
AND HOW I CAN OVERCOME THEM:
_____
_____
_____
_____

WAYS I'D LIKE TO CONNECT MORE:
_____
_____
_____
_____
_____

RECORD

DATE ___/___/___

MY GOALS FOR MEANINGFUL CONNECTIONS TODAY:

- [ ] _____
- [ ] _____
- [ ] _____

PEOPLE I'D LIKE TO CONNECT WITH:
_____
_____

WAYS TO STRENGTHEN MY RELATIONSHIPS:
_____
_____

WAYS I CONNECTED WITH OTHERS TODAY:

- [ ] CALLED A FRIEND
- [ ] ENCOURAGED SOMEONE
- [ ] ASKED FOR HELP OR ADVICE
- [ ] PLANNED ONE-ON-ONE TIME
- [ ] PRACTICED ACTIVE LISTENING
- [ ] EXPRESSED MY GRATITUDE TO SOMEONE ELSE
- [ ] SPENT QUALITY TIME WITH A FRIEND OR FAMILY MEMBER
- [ ] HELPED SOMEONE
- [ ] SHARED SOMETHING PERSONAL ABOUT MYSELF
- [ ] PRACTICED VULNERABILITY WITH A TRUSTED FRIEND
- [ ] SHARED A LAUGH
- [ ] TALKED TO SOMEONE NEW
- [ ] COMPLIMENTED SOMEONE
- [ ] COMPLETED A SHARED ACTIVITY
- [ ] NOTED SOMEONE ELSE'S MEANINGFUL DATE, EVENT, OR INTEREST I'D LIKE TO REMEMBER
- [ ] LET SOMEONE KNOW I WAS THINKING OF THEM
- [ ] PRACTICED BEING MORE PRESENT WITH OTHERS
- [ ] SHARED A STORY
- [ ] WROTE A PERSONAL NOTE OR TEXT

REFLECT

HOW I'D RATE MY FEELING OF CONNECTION TODAY:

| 1 | 2 | 3 | 4 | 5 | 6 | 7 | 8 | 9 | 10 |

LONELY / DISCONNECTED   HIGHLY CONNECTED

THE MOST MEANINGFUL INTERACTION
I HAD TODAY AND HOW IT MADE ME FEEL:

___

CHALLENGES TO DEVELOPING DEEPER BONDS
AND HOW I CAN OVERCOME THEM:

___

WAYS I'D LIKE TO CONNECT MORE:

RECORD

DATE ___ / ___ / ___

MY GOALS FOR MEANINGFUL CONNECTIONS TODAY:

- ☐ _____
- ☐ _____
- ☐ _____

PEOPLE I'D LIKE TO CONNECT WITH:

_____
_____

WAYS TO STRENGTHEN MY RELATIONSHIPS:

_____
_____

WAYS I CONNECTED WITH OTHERS TODAY:

- ☐ CALLED A FRIEND
- ☐ ENCOURAGED SOMEONE
- ☐ ASKED FOR HELP OR ADVICE
- ☐ PLANNED ONE-ON-ONE TIME
- ☐ PRACTICED ACTIVE LISTENING
- ☐ EXPRESSED MY GRATITUDE TO SOMEONE ELSE
- ☐ SPENT QUALITY TIME WITH A FRIEND OR FAMILY MEMBER
- ☐ HELPED SOMEONE
- ☐ SHARED SOMETHING PERSONAL ABOUT MYSELF
- ☐ PRACTICED VULNERABILITY WITH A TRUSTED FRIEND
- ☐ SHARED A LAUGH
- ☐ TALKED TO SOMEONE NEW
- ☐ COMPLIMENTED SOMEONE
- ☐ COMPLETED A SHARED ACTIVITY
- ☐ NOTED SOMEONE ELSE'S MEANINGFUL DATE, EVENT, OR INTEREST I'D LIKE TO REMEMBER
- ☐ LET SOMEONE KNOW I WAS THINKING OF THEM
- ☐ PRACTICED BEING MORE PRESENT WITH OTHERS
- ☐ SHARED A STORY
- ☐ WROTE A PERSONAL NOTE OR TEXT

REFLECT

HOW I'D RATE MY FEELING OF CONNECTION TODAY:

| 1 | 2 | 3 | 4 | 5 | 6 | 7 | 8 | 9 | 10 |

LONELY / DISCONNECTED   HIGHLY CONNECTED

THE MOST MEANINGFUL INTERACTION I HAD TODAY AND HOW IT MADE ME FEEL:

_____
_____
_____
_____
_____
_____
_____

CHALLENGES TO DEVELOPING DEEPER BONDS AND HOW I CAN OVERCOME THEM:

_____
_____
_____
_____

WAYS I'D LIKE TO CONNECT MORE:

_____
_____
_____
_____

RECORD

DATE ____/____/____

MY GOALS FOR MEANINGFUL CONNECTIONS TODAY:

☐ _____
☐ _____
☐ _____

PEOPLE I'D LIKE TO CONNECT WITH:

_____
_____

WAYS TO STRENGTHEN MY RELATIONSHIPS:

_____
_____

WAYS I CONNECTED WITH OTHERS TODAY:

☐ CALLED A FRIEND
☐ ENCOURAGED SOMEONE
☐ ASKED FOR HELP OR ADVICE
☐ PLANNED ONE-ON-ONE TIME
☐ PRACTICED ACTIVE LISTENING
☐ EXPRESSED MY GRATITUDE TO SOMEONE ELSE
☐ SPENT QUALITY TIME WITH A FRIEND OR FAMILY MEMBER
☐ HELPED SOMEONE
☐ SHARED SOMETHING PERSONAL ABOUT MYSELF
☐ PRACTICED VULNERABILITY WITH A TRUSTED FRIEND

☐ SHARED A LAUGH
☐ TALKED TO SOMEONE NEW
☐ COMPLIMENTED SOMEONE
☐ COMPLETED A SHARED ACTIVITY
☐ NOTED SOMEONE ELSE'S MEANINGFUL DATE, EVENT, OR INTEREST I'D LIKE TO REMEMBER
☐ LET SOMEONE KNOW I WAS THINKING OF THEM
☐ PRACTICED BEING MORE PRESENT WITH OTHERS
☐ SHARED A STORY
☐ WROTE A PERSONAL NOTE OR TEXT

REFLECT

HOW I'D RATE MY FEELING OF CONNECTION TODAY:

| 1 | 2 | 3 | 4 | 5 | 6 | 7 | 8 | 9 | 10 |

LONELY / DISCONNECTED   HIGHLY CONNECTED

THE MOST MEANINGFUL INTERACTION
I HAD TODAY AND HOW IT MADE ME FEEL:

_____
_____
_____
_____
_____
_____
_____
_____

CHALLENGES TO DEVELOPING DEEPER BONDS
AND HOW I CAN OVERCOME THEM:

_____
_____
_____
_____

WAYS I'D LIKE TO CONNECT MORE:

_____
_____
_____
_____

RECORD

DATE ___/___/___

MY GOALS FOR MEANINGFUL CONNECTIONS TODAY:

- [ ] _____
- [ ] _____
- [ ] _____

PEOPLE I'D LIKE TO CONNECT WITH:

_____
_____

WAYS TO STRENGTHEN MY RELATIONSHIPS:

_____
_____

WAYS I CONNECTED WITH OTHERS TODAY:

- [ ] CALLED A FRIEND
- [ ] ENCOURAGED SOMEONE
- [ ] ASKED FOR HELP OR ADVICE
- [ ] PLANNED ONE-ON-ONE TIME
- [ ] PRACTICED ACTIVE LISTENING
- [ ] EXPRESSED MY GRATITUDE TO SOMEONE ELSE
- [ ] SPENT QUALITY TIME WITH A FRIEND OR FAMILY MEMBER
- [ ] HELPED SOMEONE
- [ ] SHARED SOMETHING PERSONAL ABOUT MYSELF
- [ ] PRACTICED VULNERABILITY WITH A TRUSTED FRIEND
- [ ] SHARED A LAUGH
- [ ] TALKED TO SOMEONE NEW
- [ ] COMPLIMENTED SOMEONE
- [ ] COMPLETED A SHARED ACTIVITY
- [ ] NOTED SOMEONE ELSE'S MEANINGFUL DATE, EVENT, OR INTEREST I'D LIKE TO REMEMBER
- [ ] LET SOMEONE KNOW I WAS THINKING OF THEM
- [ ] PRACTICED BEING MORE PRESENT WITH OTHERS
- [ ] SHARED A STORY
- [ ] WROTE A PERSONAL NOTE OR TEXT

REFLECT

HOW I'D RATE MY FEELING OF CONNECTION TODAY:

| 1 | 2 | 3 | 4 | 5 | 6 | 7 | 8 | 9 | 10 |

LONELY / DISCONNECTED   HIGHLY CONNECTED

THE MOST MEANINGFUL INTERACTION I HAD TODAY AND HOW IT MADE ME FEEL:

_____
_____
_____
_____
_____
_____
_____
_____

CHALLENGES TO DEVELOPING DEEPER BONDS AND HOW I CAN OVERCOME THEM:

_____
_____
_____
_____

WAYS I'D LIKE TO CONNECT MORE:

_____
_____
_____
_____

RECORD

DATE ___/___/___

MY GOALS FOR MEANINGFUL CONNECTIONS TODAY:

- ☐ _____
- ☐ _____
- ☐ _____

PEOPLE I'D LIKE TO CONNECT WITH:

_____
_____

WAYS TO STRENGTHEN MY RELATIONSHIPS:

_____
_____

WAYS I CONNECTED WITH OTHERS TODAY:

- ☐ CALLED A FRIEND
- ☐ ENCOURAGED SOMEONE
- ☐ ASKED FOR HELP OR ADVICE
- ☐ PLANNED ONE-ON-ONE TIME
- ☐ PRACTICED ACTIVE LISTENING
- ☐ EXPRESSED MY GRATITUDE TO SOMEONE ELSE
- ☐ SPENT QUALITY TIME WITH A FRIEND OR FAMILY MEMBER
- ☐ HELPED SOMEONE
- ☐ SHARED SOMETHING PERSONAL ABOUT MYSELF
- ☐ PRACTICED VULNERABILITY WITH A TRUSTED FRIEND
- ☐ SHARED A LAUGH
- ☐ TALKED TO SOMEONE NEW
- ☐ COMPLIMENTED SOMEONE
- ☐ COMPLETED A SHARED ACTIVITY
- ☐ NOTED SOMEONE ELSE'S MEANINGFUL DATE, EVENT, OR INTEREST I'D LIKE TO REMEMBER
- ☐ LET SOMEONE KNOW I WAS THINKING OF THEM
- ☐ PRACTICED BEING MORE PRESENT WITH OTHERS
- ☐ SHARED A STORY
- ☐ WROTE A PERSONAL NOTE OR TEXT

REFLECT

HOW I'D RATE MY FEELING OF CONNECTION TODAY:

| 1 | 2 | 3 | 4 | 5 | 6 | 7 | 8 | 9 | 10 |

LONELY / DISCONNECTED   HIGHLY CONNECTED

THE MOST MEANINGFUL INTERACTION
I HAD TODAY AND HOW IT MADE ME FEEL:

_____
_____
_____
_____
_____
_____
_____
_____

CHALLENGES TO DEVELOPING DEEPER BONDS
AND HOW I CAN OVERCOME THEM:

_____
_____
_____
_____

WAYS I'D LIKE TO CONNECT MORE:

_____
_____
_____
_____

RECORD

DATE ___/___/___

MY GOALS FOR MEANINGFUL CONNECTIONS TODAY:

☐ _____
☐ _____
☐ _____

PEOPLE I'D LIKE TO CONNECT WITH:

_____
_____

WAYS TO STRENGTHEN MY RELATIONSHIPS:

_____
_____

WAYS I CONNECTED WITH OTHERS TODAY:

☐ CALLED A FRIEND
☐ ENCOURAGED SOMEONE
☐ ASKED FOR HELP OR ADVICE
☐ PLANNED ONE-ON-ONE TIME
☐ PRACTICED ACTIVE LISTENING
☐ EXPRESSED MY GRATITUDE TO SOMEONE ELSE
☐ SPENT QUALITY TIME WITH A FRIEND OR FAMILY MEMBER
☐ HELPED SOMEONE
☐ SHARED SOMETHING PERSONAL ABOUT MYSELF
☐ PRACTICED VULNERABILITY WITH A TRUSTED FRIEND
☐ SHARED A LAUGH
☐ TALKED TO SOMEONE NEW
☐ COMPLIMENTED SOMEONE
☐ COMPLETED A SHARED ACTIVITY
☐ NOTED SOMEONE ELSE'S MEANINGFUL DATE, EVENT, OR INTEREST I'D LIKE TO REMEMBER
☐ LET SOMEONE KNOW I WAS THINKING OF THEM
☐ PRACTICED BEING MORE PRESENT WITH OTHERS
☐ SHARED A STORY
☐ WROTE A PERSONAL NOTE OR TEXT

REFLECT

HOW I'D RATE MY FEELING OF CONNECTION TODAY:

| 1 | 2 | 3 | 4 | 5 | 6 | 7 | 8 | 9 | 10 |

LONELY / DISCONNECTED   HIGHLY CONNECTED

THE MOST MEANINGFUL INTERACTION
I HAD TODAY AND HOW IT MADE ME FEEL:
_____
_____
_____
_____
_____
_____
_____
_____

CHALLENGES TO DEVELOPING DEEPER BONDS
AND HOW I CAN OVERCOME THEM:
_____
_____
_____
_____

WAYS I'D LIKE TO CONNECT MORE:
_____
_____
_____
_____

RECORD

DATE ___/___/___

MY GOALS FOR MEANINGFUL CONNECTIONS TODAY:

- ☐ _____
- ☐ _____
- ☐ _____

PEOPLE I'D LIKE TO CONNECT WITH:
_____
_____

WAYS TO STRENGTHEN MY RELATIONSHIPS:
_____
_____

WAYS I CONNECTED WITH OTHERS TODAY:

- ☐ CALLED A FRIEND
- ☐ ENCOURAGED SOMEONE
- ☐ ASKED FOR HELP OR ADVICE
- ☐ PLANNED ONE-ON-ONE TIME
- ☐ PRACTICED ACTIVE LISTENING
- ☐ EXPRESSED MY GRATITUDE TO SOMEONE ELSE
- ☐ SPENT QUALITY TIME WITH A FRIEND OR FAMILY MEMBER
- ☐ HELPED SOMEONE
- ☐ SHARED SOMETHING PERSONAL ABOUT MYSELF
- ☐ PRACTICED VULNERABILITY WITH A TRUSTED FRIEND
- ☐ SHARED A LAUGH
- ☐ TALKED TO SOMEONE NEW
- ☐ COMPLIMENTED SOMEONE
- ☐ COMPLETED A SHARED ACTIVITY
- ☐ NOTED SOMEONE ELSE'S MEANINGFUL DATE, EVENT, OR INTEREST I'D LIKE TO REMEMBER
- ☐ LET SOMEONE KNOW I WAS THINKING OF THEM
- ☐ PRACTICED BEING MORE PRESENT WITH OTHERS
- ☐ SHARED A STORY
- ☐ WROTE A PERSONAL NOTE OR TEXT

REFLECT

HOW I'D RATE MY FEELING OF CONNECTION TODAY:

| 1 | 2 | 3 | 4 | 5 | 6 | 7 | 8 | 9 | 10 |

LONELY / DISCONNECTED   HIGHLY CONNECTED

THE MOST MEANINGFUL INTERACTION
I HAD TODAY AND HOW IT MADE ME FEEL:
_____
_____
_____
_____
_____
_____
_____

CHALLENGES TO DEVELOPING DEEPER BONDS
AND HOW I CAN OVERCOME THEM:
_____
_____
_____
_____

WAYS I'D LIKE TO CONNECT MORE:
_____
_____
_____
_____

RECORD

DATE ___/___/___

MY GOALS FOR MEANINGFUL CONNECTIONS TODAY:

☐ _____
☐ _____
☐ _____

PEOPLE I'D LIKE TO CONNECT WITH:

_____
_____

WAYS TO STRENGTHEN MY RELATIONSHIPS:

_____
_____

WAYS I CONNECTED WITH OTHERS TODAY:

- ☐ CALLED A FRIEND
- ☐ ENCOURAGED SOMEONE
- ☐ ASKED FOR HELP OR ADVICE
- ☐ PLANNED ONE-ON-ONE TIME
- ☐ PRACTICED ACTIVE LISTENING
- ☐ EXPRESSED MY GRATITUDE TO SOMEONE ELSE
- ☐ SPENT QUALITY TIME WITH A FRIEND OR FAMILY MEMBER
- ☐ HELPED SOMEONE
- ☐ SHARED SOMETHING PERSONAL ABOUT MYSELF
- ☐ PRACTICED VULNERABILITY WITH A TRUSTED FRIEND
- ☐ SHARED A LAUGH
- ☐ TALKED TO SOMEONE NEW
- ☐ COMPLIMENTED SOMEONE
- ☐ COMPLETED A SHARED ACTIVITY
- ☐ NOTED SOMEONE ELSE'S MEANINGFUL DATE, EVENT, OR INTEREST I'D LIKE TO REMEMBER
- ☐ LET SOMEONE KNOW I WAS THINKING OF THEM
- ☐ PRACTICED BEING MORE PRESENT WITH OTHERS
- ☐ SHARED A STORY
- ☐ WROTE A PERSONAL NOTE OR TEXT

REFLECT

HOW I'D RATE MY FEELING OF CONNECTION TODAY:

| 1 | 2 | 3 | 4 | 5 | 6 | 7 | 8 | 9 | 10 |

LONELY / DISCONNECTED   HIGHLY CONNECTED

THE MOST MEANINGFUL INTERACTION
I HAD TODAY AND HOW IT MADE ME FEEL:

_____
_____
_____
_____
_____
_____
_____

CHALLENGES TO DEVELOPING DEEPER BONDS
AND HOW I CAN OVERCOME THEM:

_____
_____
_____
_____

WAYS I'D LIKE TO CONNECT MORE:

_____
_____
_____
_____

RECORD

DATE ___/___/___

MY GOALS FOR MEANINGFUL CONNECTIONS TODAY:

- ☐ _____
- ☐ _____
- ☐ _____

PEOPLE I'D LIKE TO CONNECT WITH:

_____

_____

WAYS TO STRENGTHEN MY RELATIONSHIPS:

_____

_____

WAYS I CONNECTED WITH OTHERS TODAY:

- ☐ CALLED A FRIEND
- ☐ ENCOURAGED SOMEONE
- ☐ ASKED FOR HELP OR ADVICE
- ☐ PLANNED ONE-ON-ONE TIME
- ☐ PRACTICED ACTIVE LISTENING
- ☐ EXPRESSED MY GRATITUDE TO SOMEONE ELSE
- ☐ SPENT QUALITY TIME WITH A FRIEND OR FAMILY MEMBER
- ☐ HELPED SOMEONE
- ☐ SHARED SOMETHING PERSONAL ABOUT MYSELF
- ☐ PRACTICED VULNERABILITY WITH A TRUSTED FRIEND
- ☐ SHARED A LAUGH
- ☐ TALKED TO SOMEONE NEW
- ☐ COMPLIMENTED SOMEONE
- ☐ COMPLETED A SHARED ACTIVITY
- ☐ NOTED SOMEONE ELSE'S MEANINGFUL DATE, EVENT, OR INTEREST I'D LIKE TO REMEMBER
- ☐ LET SOMEONE KNOW I WAS THINKING OF THEM
- ☐ PRACTICED BEING MORE PRESENT WITH OTHERS
- ☐ SHARED A STORY
- ☐ WROTE A PERSONAL NOTE OR TEXT

REFLECT

HOW I'D RATE MY FEELING OF CONNECTION TODAY:

| 1 | 2 | 3 | 4 | 5 | 6 | 7 | 8 | 9 | 10 |

LONELY / DISCONNECTED   HIGHLY CONNECTED

THE MOST MEANINGFUL INTERACTION
I HAD TODAY AND HOW IT MADE ME FEEL:

_____
_____
_____
_____
_____
_____
_____
_____

CHALLENGES TO DEVELOPING DEEPER BONDS
AND HOW I CAN OVERCOME THEM:

_____
_____
_____
_____

WAYS I'D LIKE TO CONNECT MORE:

_____
_____
_____
_____

RECORD

DATE ___/___/___

MY GOALS FOR MEANINGFUL CONNECTIONS TODAY:

- [ ] _____
- [ ] _____
- [ ] _____

PEOPLE I'D LIKE TO CONNECT WITH:

_____
_____

WAYS TO STRENGTHEN MY RELATIONSHIPS:

_____
_____

WAYS I CONNECTED WITH OTHERS TODAY:

- [ ] CALLED A FRIEND
- [ ] ENCOURAGED SOMEONE
- [ ] ASKED FOR HELP OR ADVICE
- [ ] PLANNED ONE-ON-ONE TIME
- [ ] PRACTICED ACTIVE LISTENING
- [ ] EXPRESSED MY GRATITUDE TO SOMEONE ELSE
- [ ] SPENT QUALITY TIME WITH A FRIEND OR FAMILY MEMBER
- [ ] HELPED SOMEONE
- [ ] SHARED SOMETHING PERSONAL ABOUT MYSELF
- [ ] PRACTICED VULNERABILITY WITH A TRUSTED FRIEND
- [ ] SHARED A LAUGH
- [ ] TALKED TO SOMEONE NEW
- [ ] COMPLIMENTED SOMEONE
- [ ] COMPLETED A SHARED ACTIVITY
- [ ] NOTED SOMEONE ELSE'S MEANINGFUL DATE, EVENT, OR INTEREST I'D LIKE TO REMEMBER
- [ ] LET SOMEONE KNOW I WAS THINKING OF THEM
- [ ] PRACTICED BEING MORE PRESENT WITH OTHERS
- [ ] SHARED A STORY
- [ ] WROTE A PERSONAL NOTE OR TEXT

REFLECT

HOW I'D RATE MY FEELING OF CONNECTION TODAY:

| 1 | 2 | 3 | 4 | 5 | 6 | 7 | 8 | 9 | 10 |

LONELY / DISCONNECTED   HIGHLY CONNECTED

THE MOST MEANINGFUL INTERACTION
I HAD TODAY AND HOW IT MADE ME FEEL:

_____
_____
_____
_____
_____
_____
_____
_____

CHALLENGES TO DEVELOPING DEEPER BONDS
AND HOW I CAN OVERCOME THEM:

_____
_____
_____

WAYS I'D LIKE TO CONNECT MORE:

_____
_____
_____
_____

RECORD

DATE ___/___/___

MY GOALS FOR MEANINGFUL CONNECTIONS TODAY:

☐ _____
☐ _____
☐ _____

PEOPLE I'D LIKE TO CONNECT WITH:

_____
_____

WAYS TO STRENGTHEN MY RELATIONSHIPS:

_____
_____

WAYS I CONNECTED WITH OTHERS TODAY:

☐ CALLED A FRIEND
☐ ENCOURAGED SOMEONE
☐ ASKED FOR HELP OR ADVICE
☐ PLANNED ONE-ON-ONE TIME
☐ PRACTICED ACTIVE LISTENING
☐ EXPRESSED MY GRATITUDE TO SOMEONE ELSE
☐ SPENT QUALITY TIME WITH A FRIEND OR FAMILY MEMBER
☐ HELPED SOMEONE
☐ SHARED SOMETHING PERSONAL ABOUT MYSELF
☐ PRACTICED VULNERABILITY WITH A TRUSTED FRIEND

☐ SHARED A LAUGH
☐ TALKED TO SOMEONE NEW
☐ COMPLIMENTED SOMEONE
☐ COMPLETED A SHARED ACTIVITY
☐ NOTED SOMEONE ELSE'S MEANINGFUL DATE, EVENT, OR INTEREST I'D LIKE TO REMEMBER
☐ LET SOMEONE KNOW I WAS THINKING OF THEM
☐ PRACTICED BEING MORE PRESENT WITH OTHERS
☐ SHARED A STORY
☐ WROTE A PERSONAL NOTE OR TEXT

REFLECT

HOW I'D RATE MY FEELING OF CONNECTION TODAY:

| 1 | 2 | 3 | 4 | 5 | 6 | 7 | 8 | 9 | 10 |

LONELY / DISCONNECTED   HIGHLY CONNECTED

THE MOST MEANINGFUL INTERACTION
I HAD TODAY AND HOW IT MADE ME FEEL:

_____
_____
_____
_____
_____
_____
_____

CHALLENGES TO DEVELOPING DEEPER BONDS
AND HOW I CAN OVERCOME THEM:

_____
_____
_____
_____

WAYS I'D LIKE TO CONNECT MORE:

_____
_____
_____
_____
_____

RECORD

DATE ___/___/___

MY GOALS FOR MEANINGFUL CONNECTIONS TODAY:

☐ _____
☐ _____
☐ _____

PEOPLE I'D LIKE TO CONNECT WITH:

_____
_____

WAYS TO STRENGTHEN MY RELATIONSHIPS:

_____
_____

WAYS I CONNECTED WITH OTHERS TODAY:

- ☐ CALLED A FRIEND
- ☐ ENCOURAGED SOMEONE
- ☐ ASKED FOR HELP OR ADVICE
- ☐ PLANNED ONE-ON-ONE TIME
- ☐ PRACTICED ACTIVE LISTENING
- ☐ EXPRESSED MY GRATITUDE TO SOMEONE ELSE
- ☐ SPENT QUALITY TIME WITH A FRIEND OR FAMILY MEMBER
- ☐ HELPED SOMEONE
- ☐ SHARED SOMETHING PERSONAL ABOUT MYSELF
- ☐ PRACTICED VULNERABILITY WITH A TRUSTED FRIEND
- ☐ SHARED A LAUGH
- ☐ TALKED TO SOMEONE NEW
- ☐ COMPLIMENTED SOMEONE
- ☐ COMPLETED A SHARED ACTIVITY
- ☐ NOTED SOMEONE ELSE'S MEANINGFUL DATE, EVENT, OR INTEREST I'D LIKE TO REMEMBER
- ☐ LET SOMEONE KNOW I WAS THINKING OF THEM
- ☐ PRACTICED BEING MORE PRESENT WITH OTHERS
- ☐ SHARED A STORY
- ☐ WROTE A PERSONAL NOTE OR TEXT

REFLECT

HOW I'D RATE MY FEELING OF CONNECTION TODAY:

| 1 | 2 | 3 | 4 | 5 | 6 | 7 | 8 | 9 | 10 |

LONELY / DISCONNECTED   HIGHLY CONNECTED

THE MOST MEANINGFUL INTERACTION
I HAD TODAY AND HOW IT MADE ME FEEL:
_____
_____
_____
_____
_____
_____
_____
_____
_____

CHALLENGES TO DEVELOPING DEEPER BONDS
AND HOW I CAN OVERCOME THEM:
_____
_____
_____
_____

WAYS I'D LIKE TO CONNECT MORE:
_____
_____
_____
_____
_____

RECORD

DATE ___/___/___

MY GOALS FOR MEANINGFUL CONNECTIONS TODAY:

- ☐ _____
- ☐ _____
- ☐ _____

PEOPLE I'D LIKE TO CONNECT WITH:
_____
_____

WAYS TO STRENGTHEN MY RELATIONSHIPS:
_____
_____

WAYS I CONNECTED WITH OTHERS TODAY:

- ☐ CALLED A FRIEND
- ☐ ENCOURAGED SOMEONE
- ☐ ASKED FOR HELP OR ADVICE
- ☐ PLANNED ONE-ON-ONE TIME
- ☐ PRACTICED ACTIVE LISTENING
- ☐ EXPRESSED MY GRATITUDE TO SOMEONE ELSE
- ☐ SPENT QUALITY TIME WITH A FRIEND OR FAMILY MEMBER
- ☐ HELPED SOMEONE
- ☐ SHARED SOMETHING PERSONAL ABOUT MYSELF
- ☐ PRACTICED VULNERABILITY WITH A TRUSTED FRIEND

- ☐ SHARED A LAUGH
- ☐ TALKED TO SOMEONE NEW
- ☐ COMPLIMENTED SOMEONE
- ☐ COMPLETED A SHARED ACTIVITY
- ☐ NOTED SOMEONE ELSE'S MEANINGFUL DATE, EVENT, OR INTEREST I'D LIKE TO REMEMBER
- ☐ LET SOMEONE KNOW I WAS THINKING OF THEM
- ☐ PRACTICED BEING MORE PRESENT WITH OTHERS
- ☐ SHARED A STORY
- ☐ WROTE A PERSONAL NOTE OR TEXT

REFLECT

HOW I'D RATE MY FEELING OF CONNECTION TODAY:

| 1 | 2 | 3 | 4 | 5 | 6 | 7 | 8 | 9 | 10 |

LONELY / DISCONNECTED   HIGHLY CONNECTED

THE MOST MEANINGFUL INTERACTION
I HAD TODAY AND HOW IT MADE ME FEEL:
_____
_____
_____
_____
_____
_____
_____
_____

CHALLENGES TO DEVELOPING DEEPER BONDS
AND HOW I CAN OVERCOME THEM:
_____
_____
_____
_____

WAYS I'D LIKE TO CONNECT MORE:
_____
_____
_____
_____
_____

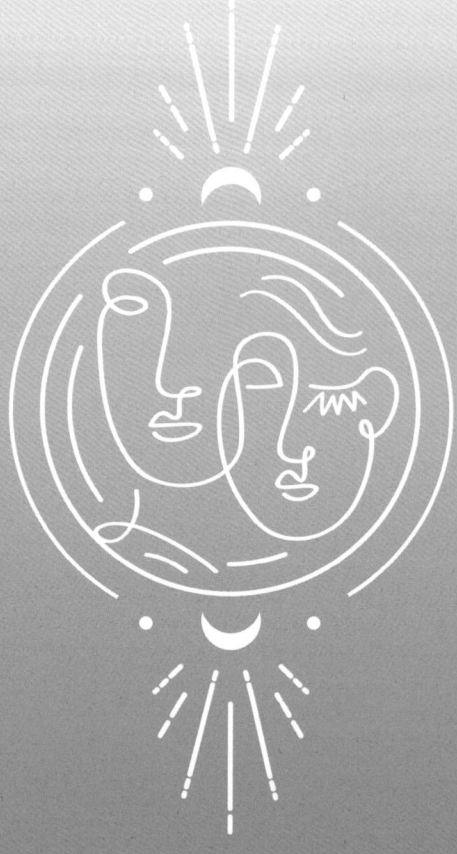

INSIGHTS
A Mandala Journal

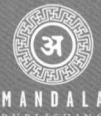

MANDALA
PUBLISHING

www.mandalaearth.com

Copyright © 2021 Mandala Publishing. All rights reserved.
MANUFACTURED IN CHINA
10 9 8 7 6 5 4 3 2 1

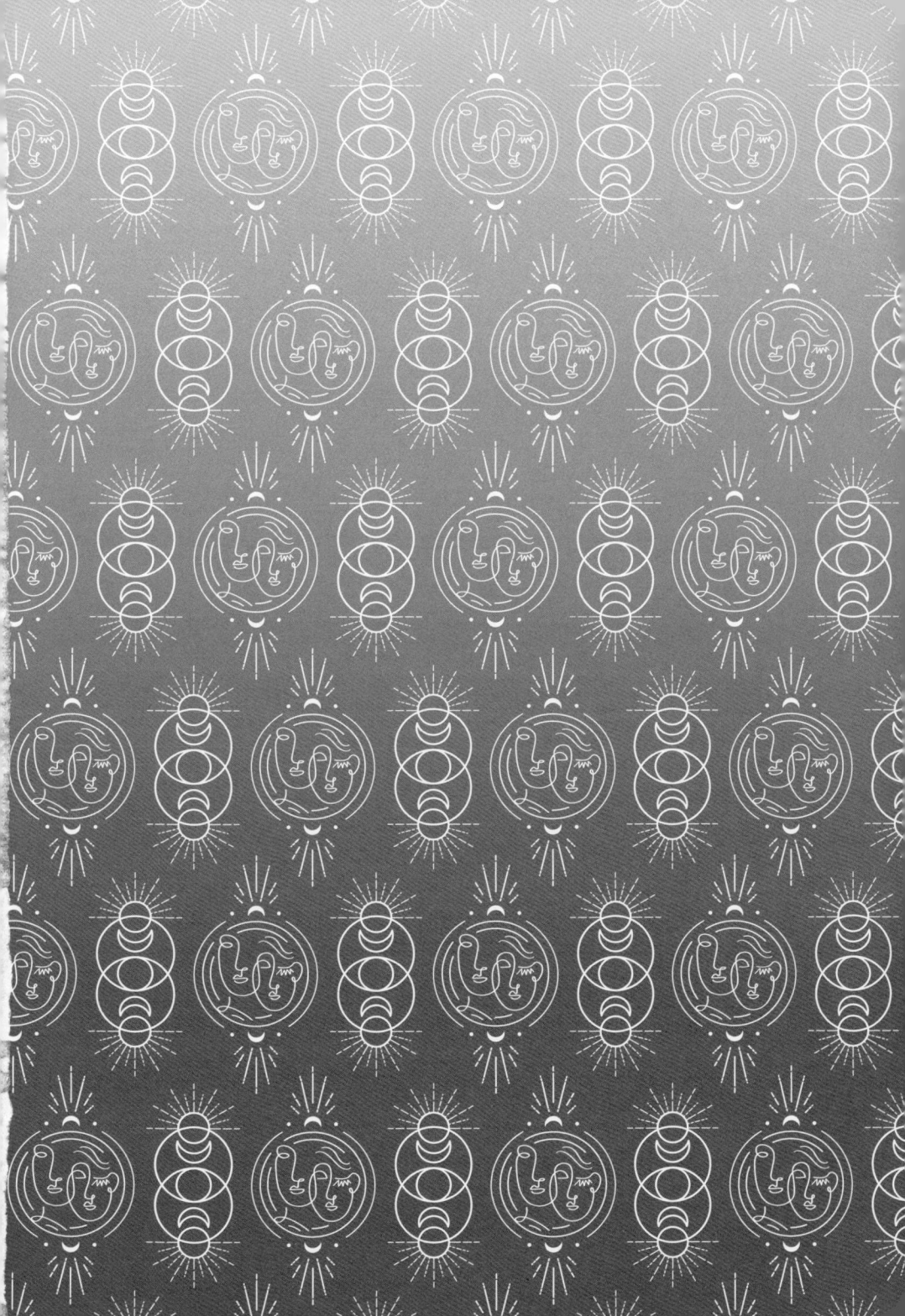

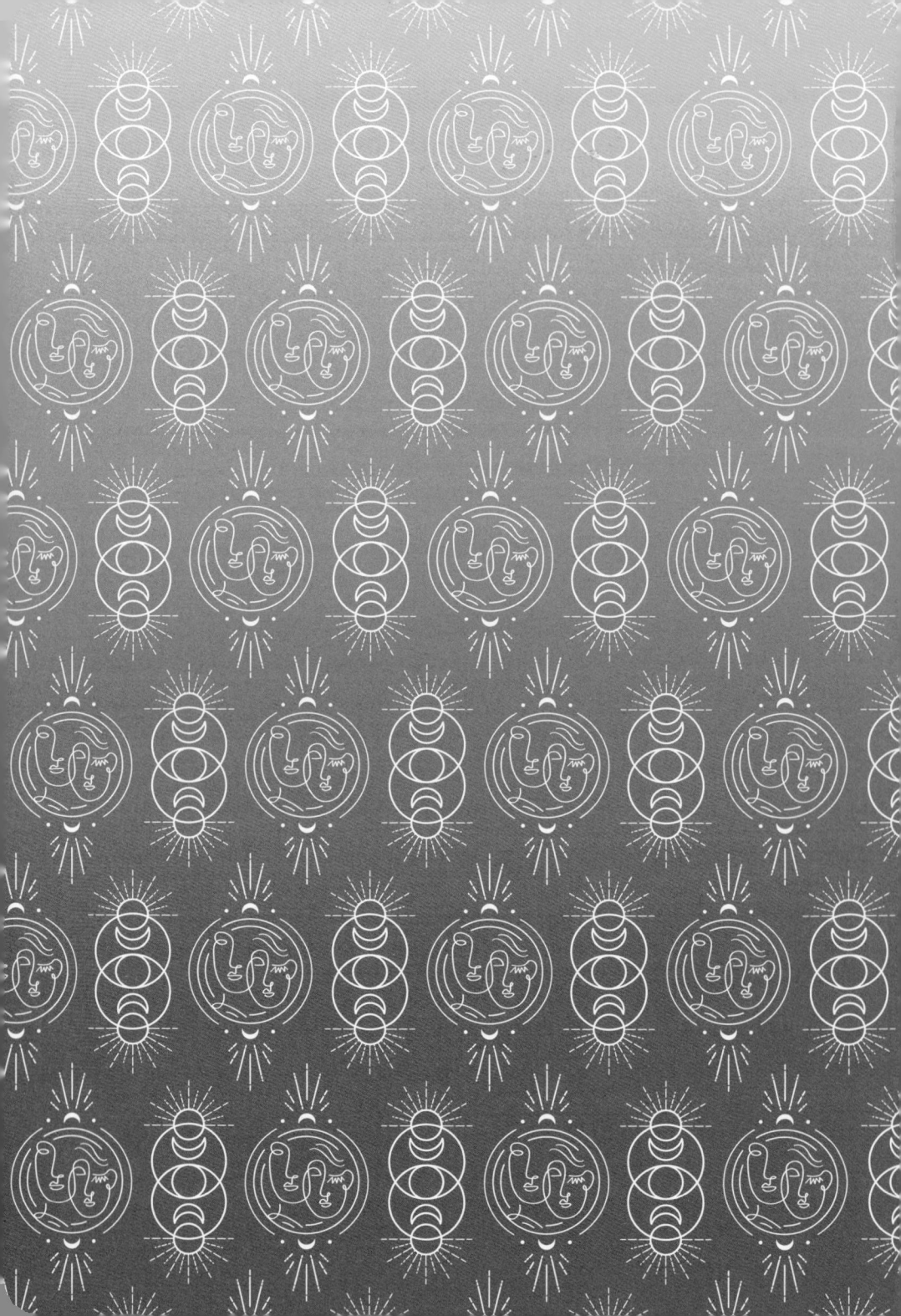